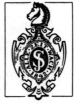

Clinical Practice in Urology

Series Editor: Geoffrey D. Chisholm

The Pharmacology of the Urinary Tract

Edited by
Marco Caine

With 27 Figures

Springer-Verlag
Berlin Heidelberg New York Tokyo
1984

Marco Caine, MS, FRCS, FACS
Professor of Urology, Hebrew University, Jerusalem; and Director,
Department of Urology, Hadassah University Hospital, Jerusalem,
Israel

Series Editor
Geoffrey D. Chisholm, ChM, FRCS, FRCSEd Professor of Surgery,
University of Edinburgh; and Consultant Urological Surgeon,
Western General Hospital, Edinburgh, Scotland

ISBN–13:978–1–4471–1361–4   e–ISBN–13:978–1–4471–1359–1
DOI: 10.1007/978–1–4471–1359–1

Library of Congress Cataloging in Publication Data
Main entry under title:
The Pharmacology of the urinary tract.
(Clinical practice in urology)
Includes bibliographies and index. 1. Urinary organs – Diseases – Chemotheropy. 2.
Urinary organs – Effect of drugs on. I. Caine, Marco, 1923- . II. Series. [DNLM: 1.
Urinary Tract – drug effects. 2. Urologic Diseases – drug therapy. WJ 166
P536]   RC900.5.P45   1984   616.6′061   84-13988
ISBN–13:978–1–4471–1361–4 (U.S.)

Phototypeset by Input Typesetting Ltd London SW19 8DR

2128/3916–543210

Series Editor's Foreword

The interface between the urologist and other disciplines in medicine continues to increase as the character of urology continues to change. Urologists have, for example, developed strong links with microbiologists over mutual problems of infection in the urinary tract, urologists have been involved in the development of modern management of renal disease and especially renal failure, indeed even before the subject of nephrology had been defined. Similarly the links between endocrinology and infertility and more recently links between imaging and urology have led to the mutual benefit of these subjects and certainly to better patient care.

The Pharmacology of the urinary tract has proved to be a difficult area of study. Slowly but progressively it has become evident that this is an area of great potential for urologists. Our patients have a range of problems where non-surgical management would be ideal but finding the right drug for the right condition has remained an elusive task. Many of the earlier trials showed an impressive placebo-response rate and emphasised the need for well planned controlled clinical trials. The place of such trials in the evaluation of new treatments for urinary symptoms is now unchallenged and uncontrolled data are of little value.

This book represents a skillful combination of background information and its clinical application. The review of the pharmacokinetics of the various groups of drugs provides a very useful background to both the use of current drugs and also the prospects for the future. Without this information there is a serious risk of prescribing the wrong drug in the wrong dose or prescribing drugs of similar mechanism of action when what is needed is an entirely different approach. Professor Caine has assembled a group of well known experts in this field and their collective wisdom should enable the urologist to use these pharmacological agents to their best advantage in clinical practice.

Edinburgh July 1984   Geoffrey Chisholm

Preface

It is an interesting indication of the scope of modern urology that in a series of books devoted to clinical practice in urology, and directed particularly towards the practising urologist, it should be thought desirable to devote a volume to the pharmacology of the urinary tract. This reflects the fact that the modern urological surgeon is concerned not only with the structural changes produced by disease, but also with physiological mechanisms and the disturbances of function met with in both the upper and the lower urinary tracts.

Since the functioning of the urinary tract can often be modified by pharmacological agents, it behoves the urologist to be fully conversant with the various drugs that can act upon it. It must be remembered that, in addition to the armamentarium used with the specific aim of modifying urinary tract function, the urologist will not infrequently encounter drugs given to a patient for other purposes, but which incidentally produce unintentional side-effects on the urinary tract. It is partly with this consideration in mind that the list of common proprietary names under which the urologist may meet the drugs mentioned in the text, together with their official equivalents, is appended.

The study of the pharmacology of the urinary tract is a very active field of research, and hardly a month goes by without a number of papers on the subject appearing in the urological literature. This means that no book can hope to keep abreast of the work being done, or to be completely up to date by the time it appears in print. None the less, the urologist is frequently confronted by fresh developments and new preparations, which it is necessary for him to be able to assess. Accordingly, although the primary aim of this book is to give the reader an up-to-date account of the clinical uses and applications of existing drugs, it was felt to be equally important to include a review of the underlying principles relating to the modes of action of the different groups of agents. To this end the text has been divided into two parts, the first dealing with the principles of urinary tract pharmacology and the second with the use of pharmacological agents in urinary tract disorders. It is hoped that this will not only give the reader an understanding of the modes of action of the various drugs in use today, thus enabling him to employ them in a fully informed and logical manner, but also enable him to assess for himself future developments and proposed drugs as they appear in the literature or on the market. This plan inevitably results in a certain degree of overlap and duplication of material in the different chapters. However, having regard to the fact that chapters in a book such as this are frequently read independently of each other, and in order to ensure maximum clarity in each, this has been considered to be justified.

As will be seen, the urologist frequently encounters a variety of drugs which can produce very similar or identical effects on the urinary tract, and the decision as to which to use in a given case may be difficult. The present authors, all of whom are well-known authorities in their fields have in addition to giving their own views, generally provided surveys of the background information and experimental and clinical experience with the different agents. These should assist the reader to make up his or her own mind as to which drug or combination of drugs to use in a particular patient.

Jerusalem, 1984   Marco Caine

Acknowledgements

In concluding, I should like to express my thanks to all those who have helped so much in bringing this book to fruition. Firstly, my sincere thanks to the colleagues who have joined me and contributed so generously of their personal expertise, despite the heavy demands already made on their time. The wisdom and experience of both Geoffrey Chisholm and Michael Jackson have been unfailing sources of help and encouragement, and I am most grateful for their constant courtesy and patience. It is a pleasure to be able to thank my secretary, Mrs Haya Medalia, for her indefatigable patience and good humour in the preparation of this manuscript. Finally, I should like to dedicate this book to my wife Dolly, as a small recompense for the many hours she has had to put up with my absence as a result of the demands of our profession.

Contents

PART II. USE OF PHARMACOLOGICAL AGENTS IN
URINARY TRACT DISORDERS

Contributors

Saul Boyarsky, Washington University School of Medicine, Division of Urology/216 Wohl Hospital, 4960 Audubon Avenue, St Louis, Missouri 63110, USA

Marco Caine, Professor of Urology, Hadassah Medical Organisation, Hadassah University Hospital Kiryat Hadassah, POB 12000, Jerusalem 91 120, Israel

Ananias C. Diokno, Professor of Urology, Section of Urology, Department of Surgery, University of Michigan, Ann Arbor, Michigan 48109, USA

Amos Shapiro, Assistant Surgeon, Department of Urology, Hadassah University Hospital, POB 12000, Jerusalem 91 120, Israel

L. Paul Sonda, Assistant Professor, Section of Urology, Department of Surgery, University of Michigan, Ann Arbor, Michigan 48109, USA

Alan J. Wein, Chairman, Division of Urology, University of Pennsylvania School of Medicine, 5 Silverstein, 3400 Spruce Street, Philadelphia, Pennsylvania 19104, USA

PART I

PRINCIPLES OF URINARY TRACT PHARMACOLOGY

Introduction

The essential functions of the urinary tract, from the collecting system of the kidneys onwards, are those of transport and storage of the urine until it eventually leaves the body. These functions depend upon the activity of the muscle in the walls of the urinary tract, and for practical purposes most of the pharmacology of the urinary tract is concerned with the actions of pharmacological agents upon this muscle, which results in modifications of its activity and tone. By far the greater part of the musculature is visceral smooth muscle, and therefore the emphasis is upon smooth muscle pharmacology. In addition, however, there is a striated muscle component of considerable importance associated with the outflow tract from the bladder, and the relevant effects of pharmacological agents upon this tissue are dealt with specifically in Chap. 3.

The tone and activity of the smooth muscle of the urinary tract, as is the case elsewhere in the body, are largely under the control of the autonomic nervous system, and it is possible for pharmacological agents to affect the urinary system by acting on or via this control system, by acting directly on the muscle itself, or by a combination of both actions. Before dealing with the autonomic nervous supply to the urinary tract, and the effects of drugs upon this or upon the smooth muscle fibres, it is advisable to recall briefly some of the salient features of the intracellular biological processes associated with smooth muscle activity.

Biology of Smooth Muscle

The ability of the smooth muscle cell to contract is due to the presence therein of two contractile proteins, actin and myosin, distributed in the form of longitudinal microfilaments. The actual contraction of the cell is produced by a sliding of the thin actin filaments over the thick myosin filaments as a result of their activation. The energy necessary for this is derived from the hydrolysis of adenosine triphosphate (ATP). The activation is brought about by an increase of ionised calcium in the cell, which in turn may result either from an increased entry of calcium ions into the cell due to changes in the permeability of the cell membrane, or from mobilisation of the ions from calcium stores already existing within the cell. There is now good evidence that the calcium ions themselves do not have a direct action, but that they are first bound to calmodulin, a widely distributed protein found in most nucleated cells. This calcium–calmodulin complex can activate a number of enzymes, including the one relevant to this context which is known as the myosin light-chain kinase. It is believed that this enzyme catalyses the phosphorylation of myosin and activates the ATPase in it; this in turn hydrolyses the ATP and thus releases the energy needed for muscle contraction.

Although the exact modes of action at a molecular biological level of most of the pharmacological agents are not yet fully understood, it will be seen below that in some cases enough is known to afford a rational explanation of their effects in terms of the modification of certain of the factors concerned with smooth muscle activation outlined above.

Chapter 1

The Autonomic Pharmacology of the Urinary Tract

Marco Caine

Autonomic Control of Smooth Muscle

In order logically to understand the actions of the many pharmacological agents in use today which produce their effects on the urinary musculature via its autonomic control, it is desirable first of all to give a brief review of present-day thinking concerning the structure and functions of the autonomic nervous system in relation to the urinary tract.

Structure of the Autonomic System

Both the sympathetic and the parasympathetic divisions of the autonomic nervous system are involved in the control of the urinary tract musculature. The relevant portion of the sympathetic outflow arises from the thoraco-lumbar (T10–L2) segments of the spinal cord, and the preganglionic neurons make synaptic connections with the postganglionic effector neurons not only in the ganglia of the paravertebral sympathetic chains, but also in more peripherally situated ganglia, or in or adjacent to the walls of the viscera themselves. The parasympathetic preganglionic neurons arise in the brain stem and the sacral cord from S2 to S4 in the human, and their synapses with the postganglionic neurons are situated mainly peripherally, in or adjacent to the end-organs. Although traditionally the paths of the sympathetic and parasympathetic systems were regarded as independent of each other, it is now realised that this is not so, and cross-connections are known to exist between the sympathetic and parasympathetic neurons at peripheral synaptic sites, particularly in the region of the bladder outlet, where they are probably of importance in relation to the coordinated activity of this region during the micturition cycle (Elbadawi and Schenk 1971). In addition, there are sympathetic receptor sites at the synapses between the pre- and postganglionic parasympathetic neurons which exert an inhibitory action on parasympathetic transmission (de Groat and Saum 1971).

Neurotransmitters

It is now generally accepted that the transmission of nerve impulses across the synaptic clefts, or between the postganglionic nerve and the effector cell, is mediated by a chemical substance referred to as a neurotransmitter. In the case of the postganglionic sympathetic nerves acting on the muscle this is noradrenaline, whereas in the case of the postganglionic parasympathetic nerve endings, and the synapses between the preganglionic and postganglionic neurons in both the parasympathetic and the sympathetic systems, the neurotransmitter is acetylcholine. As mentioned in Chap. 3, acetylcholine is also the neurotransmitter acting between the somatic motor nerve endings and striated muscle. The neurons liberating these neurotransmitter substances can be termed adrenergic (or noradrenergic) and cholinergic respectively, and it is worth noting that as acetylcholine is liberated by both the sympathetic and the parasympathetic preganglionic neurons, these terms are not synonymous with the terms sympathetic and parasympathetic (Fig. 1.1).

Production of Noradrenaline

Noradrenaline is synthesised in the adrenergic neurons themselves from tyrosine, via the intermediate stages of levodopa and dopamine (Fig.1.2), and is stored in granular vesicles within the neurons, probably in association with adenosine triphosphate (ATP). The rate-limiting stage in this biosynthesis is probably the conversion of tyrosine to levodopa catalysed by tyrosine

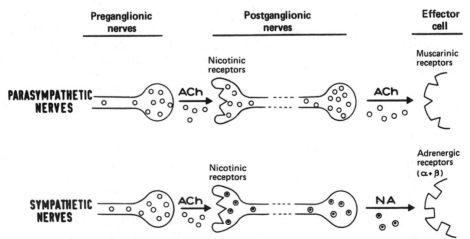

Fig. 1.1. Acetylcholine (ACh) and noradrenaline (NA) are the autonomic neurotransmitters at the sites shown.

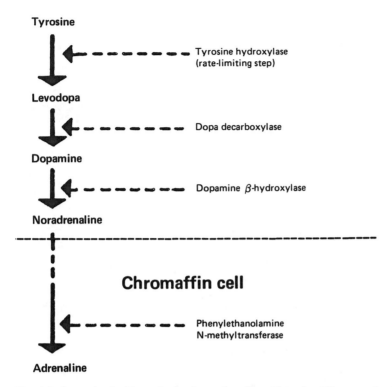

Fig. 1.2. Stages in the biosynthesis of noradrenaline. Note the different end-points in the neuron and in the chromaffin cell.

hydroxylase, which is controlled via a feedback mechanism by the amount of noradrenaline present in the neuron. These steps in the synthesis of noradrenaline are of practical importance, for as will be seen below certain of the pharmacological agents which produce an effect on the urinary tract do so by modifying some stage in this synthesis. At their terminations, the nerves undergo repeated branching resulting in a network of very fine fibres in intimate contact with the effector cells, and along these fine terminal fibres are a series of swellings or varicosities, which give the fibres a beaded appearance. There is evidence that the noradrenaline-containing vesicles formed in the cell bodies pass along the axons and are concentrated in these varicosities (Fig.1.3). On the arrival of a nerve impulse the vesicles become attached to the plasma membrane of the varicosities and discharge their contents into the synaptic cleft between the varicosity and the muscle cell, a process known as exocytosis. This process appears to be associated with an influx of calcium ions. Upon its liberation into the synaptic cleft the noradrenaline acts upon appropriate receptors, as described below (Fig.1.4). By virtue of this structural arrangement a single nerve fibre can activate a number of muscle cells, and there is also evidence that a single smooth muscle cell may be innervated by a number of nerve fibres.

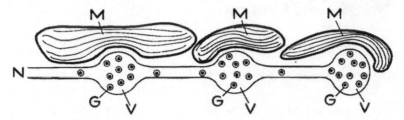

Fig. 1.3. Noradrenaline-containing vesicles concentrated in neural varicosities in intimate contact with smooth muscle cells. G, granular vesicle containing noradrenaline; M, muscle cell; N, terminal nerve fibre; V, varicosity of terminal nerve fibre.

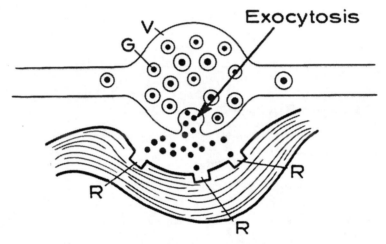

Fig. 1.4. Exocytosis liberates noradrenaline into synaptic cleft. G, granular vesicle containing noradrenaline; R, receptor on muscle cell; V, neuronal varicosity.

In addition to the local liberation of noradrenaline from the noradrenergic nerves, noradrenaline and particularly adrenaline are produced and stored in the chromaffin cells of the adrenal medulla. These adrenaline-producing cells contain an enzyme, phenylethanolamine-N-methyltransferase, which converts the noradrenaline into adrenaline (Fig.1.2). As this enzyme is not present in the noradrenergic neurons, the biosynthesis in their case does not go beyond noradrenaline. Both substances are released from the chromaffin cells as the result of stimulation by the preganglionic sympathetic neurons supplying the adrenal medulla, enter the circulation and produce their effects on the appropriate receptors throughout the body.

Inactivation of Noradrenaline

The liberated noradrenaline which is not required for activation of the effector cells is inactivated by a number of mechanisms. By far the greater part of that liberated from the neurons is re-absorbed into the nerve terminals themselves, a process called by Iversen (1965) 'uptake   . This re-uptake is prevented by degeneration of the adrenergic neurons following sympathectomy, which may afford an explanation for the supersensitivity to noradrenaline shown by denervated tissues. It is also inhibited by certain drugs, such as cocaine and imipramine. The term 'uptake 2' refers to uptake of the catecholamines by a variety of other tissues in the body, where they are deactivated by the enzymes monoamine oxidase (MAO) and catechol-O-methyltransferase (COMT). These are probably of relatively little importance in the case of the noradrenaline liberated from the neurons, but are of much greater importance in deactivating circulating catecholamines derived from the adrenal glands, or any administered parenterally (Fig.1.5). In addition, MAO is also present in the mitochondria inside the noradrenergic neurons, where it appears to be of importance in regulating the amount of noradrenaline in the neuronal cytoplasm.

Production of Acetylcholine

Acetylcholine is formed in the cholinergic neurons from a combination of acetate in the activated form of acetyl coenzyme A with choline, by means of a specific enzyme called choline acetyltransferase. This enzyme is itself produced in the cholinergic neurons, being synthesised mainly in clear vesicles at the nerve endings, and stored in them. On arrival of a nerve impulse a local change in permeability of the cell membrane to calcium ions occurs, and the contents of the vesicles are released into the synaptic cleft by exocytosis, in a similar manner to that described for the noradrenergic vesicles. At rest there is a slow random release which is insufficient to produce activation of the postsynaptic cell, but on arrival of a nerve impulse a massive discharge of acetylcholine takes place which results in the development of an action potential in the postsynaptic cell membrane, and a response in the effector cell.

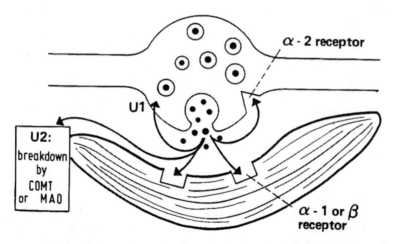

Fig. 1.5. Inactivation of noradrenaline. U_1 (uptake 1), reabsorption into nerve terminal; U_2 (uptake 2, of little importance in neural NA), uptake into tissues and deactivation by enzymes monoamine oxidase (MAO) and catechol-O-methyltransferase (COMT); α-2, presynaptic alpha receptors; α-1 or β, postsynaptic adrenergic receptors.

Inactivation of Acetylcholine

The liberated acetylcholine is extremely rapidly inactivated in situ by the enzyme acetylcholinesterase, present in the postsynaptic membranes, which hydrolyses it with the liberation of choline and acetate. Some of the choline is re-absorbed into the presynaptic nerve endings but, in contrast to noradrenaline, it appears that the acetylcholine itself is not re-absorbed into the nerve to any extent.

Autonomic Receptors

Both noradrenaline and acetylcholine are believed to produce their effects on the postsynaptic cell only after having combined with specialised sites on the cell membrane, known as receptors. These sites are relatively specific, but chemical substances other than the natural neurotransmitter may also combine with them. When these substances activate the receptors and produce a biological effect on the cell, they are known as agonists. In contrast to these agonists, there are other substances which combine with the receptors but do not produce any effect. In so doing, they can block the access of the agonists to the receptors, and are hence known as blockers or antagonists.

Adrenergic Receptors

Alpha and Beta Receptors. The sites on the effector cells with which noradrenaline combines in order to produce its action are known as adrenergic receptors or adrenoreceptors. The effect produced on the cell by noradrenergic stimulation is not uniform: in some cases a stimulating effect is obtained and in others the opposite. In 1948 Ahlquist proposed the now generally accepted concept that this variable response is due to the existence of two different types of adrenergic receptors, which he designated as alpha and beta. In most smooth muscle, including the smooth muscle of the urinary tract, stimulation of the alpha-adrenergic receptors results in excitation of the tissue, producing an increase in tone or a contraction of the muscle fibres, whereas stimulation of the beta-adrenergic receptors has an inhibitory effect, resulting in muscle relaxation and a diminished tone. An effector cell may contain either or both of these receptor types in different amounts, and it can be understood, therefore, that the net response of a tissue to noradrenergic stimulation will depend upon the type of adrenergic receptor which is present, or which is predominant. If both types of receptor are present, specific blockade of the predominant one will leave the other type to respond unopposed, and the net reaction of the tissue to adrenergic stimulation will change correspondingly.

Whether the two types of receptors are separate and independent structures, or whether they are in fact separate sites on a single structure as suggested by Belleau (1963), is not clear. What does seem to be clear, however, is that they are not fixed and immutable entities, but that changes can occur from one type to another under certain circumstances, as for example in response to temperature changes (Kunos and Nickerson 1976) or, in the case of the bladder detrusor receptors, to the presence of chronic bladder outlet obstruction (Rohner et al. 1978).

Adrenergic Receptor Subtypes. Both the alpha and beta receptors can be further divided into subtypes. In the case of the alpha receptors, in addition to those on the effector cell, which are designated as 'postsynaptic' or 'alpha-1', there appear also to be receptor sites on the nerve terminals themselves. These are designated 'presynaptic' or 'alpha-2', and they seem to be autoregulatory in nature (Berthelsen and Pettinger 1977). Stimulation of these receptors by noradrenaline present in the synaptic cleft inhibits the liberation of more noradrenaline, thus functioning as a type of negative feedback mechanism.

In the case of the beta receptors, the two types are also termed '1' and '2'. The beta-1 receptors are those involved in the positive inotropic effect produced by beta-adrenergic agonists on cardiac muscle, whereas the beta-2 receptors mediate the relaxing effects produced on vascular and bronchial smooth muscle (Lands et al. 1967). Whether or not there also exist presynaptic beta receptors comparable to the presynaptic alpha receptors, possibly facilitating noradrenaline release, is not yet established. There is some experimental evidence that the beta receptors in the urinary tract smooth muscle are of the beta-2 type (Khanna et al. 1981). These subdivisions are not only of academic interest but can also be of practical importance for, as will be seen below, certain agonists and blockers can have highly specific actions on each type of receptor.

Cholinergic Receptors

As indicated earlier, neurochemical transmission by means of acetylcholine is very widespread in the body, occurring in all the synapses between pre- and postganglionic neurons, both sympathetic and parasympathetic, between the postganglionic parasympathetic fibres and the effector cells, and at the neuromuscular junctions of striated muscle. In each instance, as is the case with noradrenaline, the acetylcholine produces its effect via an appropriate receptor. Two types of cholinergic receptors are described, according to their specific reactions to different agonists. Those on the postganglionic cell bodies, which react to acetylcholine liberated from the preganglionic neuron, are termed nicotinic, because of their response to nicotine. In low concentrations nicotine stimulates these receptors, whereas in high concentrations it blocks them. Those receptors on the effector cells which respond to acetylcholine liberated from the postganglionic autonomic nerve endings are known as muscarinic because of their response to stimulation with the fungal alkaloid muscarine. In the case of the smooth muscle of the urinary tract, stimulation of the muscarinic receptors results in an increase in tone or a contraction of the muscle fibre.

Mechanism of Receptor Action

The exact way in which each type of agonist–receptor combination produces a biological effect in the effector cell is by no means clear, although it is generally accepted that this is in some way associated with changes in the permeability of the cell membrane allowing ionic shifts. In the case of beta activity, a more detailed explanation has been put forward to account for the reduction in muscle tone. It is suggested that in this case the combination of the agonist with the receptor on the surface of the cell membrane results in activation of adenylate cyclase on the inner surface of the membrane. This, in the presence of magnesium ions, converts ATP in the cell to cyclic AMP. The

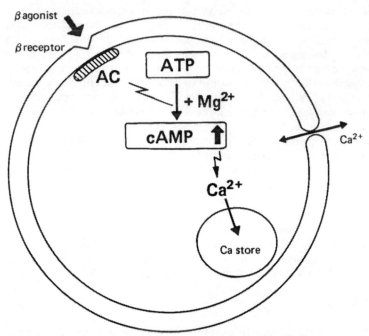

Fig. 1.6. Suggested mechanism of beta-adrenergic activation. The beta agonist stimulates the beta receptor and activates the adenylate cyclase (AC). This, in the presence of magnesium ions (Mg^{2+}) converts ATP to cyclic AMP (cAMP). The increase in the latter causes a shift of intracellular calcium ions (Ca^{2+}) into the calcium stores.

increase in cyclic AMP results in an uptake of intracellular calcium ions into the intracellular stores, thus decreasing the amount of free calcium ions in the sarcoplasm and hence reducing the activity of myosin, as explained in the Introduction (Marshall and Kroeger 1973)(Fig.1.6).

Identification of Receptors

As already indicated, the different types of autonomic receptors are not present equally in all tissues, and in recent years a considerable amount of work has been put into establishing the presence of the receptors in different organs and tissues, including their distribution throughout the urinary tract. There are a number of ways in which the presence of a given receptor can be ascertained. The most widely used is the pharmacological method, whereby the tissue's reactions to specific agonists and blockers is studied. This can be performed in vitro, in an isolated preparation of the tissue, or by an in vivo method. The latter would seem at first sight to be more physiological, but it must always be remembered that a drug administered to an intact animal can have widespread effects on many systems, and these in turn can produce secondary effects on the tissue or organ under study which may complicate and confuse the responses obtained. In vitro testing, on the other hand, although apparently less physiological, can afford a much better controlled environment in which the specific effects of agonists and blockers can be examined.

A second method of identifying receptors is by attempting to label them by means of radioactive ligands, and then to look for the radioactive sites in the tissue. This method has practical technical difficulties, largely associated with non-specific binding of the radioactive ligands to the tissues, and is still in a relatively early stage of development. A third method used is inferential, in that it is based upon identification of adrenergic and cholinergic nerve terminals; the assumption is then made that the presence of these terminals logically indicates that corresponding receptors are present. Fluorescent microscopic techniques and histochemical methods are used, which demonstrate the presence of noradrenaline granules on the one hand, or acetylcholinesterase on the other. In addition to being inferential, this method has the limitation that it cannot differentiate between the alpha- and beta-adrenergic receptors.

Distribution of Autonomic Receptors in the Urinary Tract

As a result of studies of the above types, we now possess a good knowledge of the distribution of the various autonomic receptors throughout the urinary tract (Fig. 1.7). It must always be borne in mind, though, that species differences can exist, and that the findings in an experimental animal cannot necessarily be extrapolated to the human. Luckily, a considerable amount of information derived from studies on human material obtained either at operation or at autopsy is available.

Ureter. The peristalsis of the ureter occurs independently of any nerve supply, as can be seen in the case of the transplanted kidney and ureter, but both the rate and amplitude of peristalsis can be modified by nervous influences. Both adrenergic and cholinergic terminal nerve fibres have been demonstrated in the

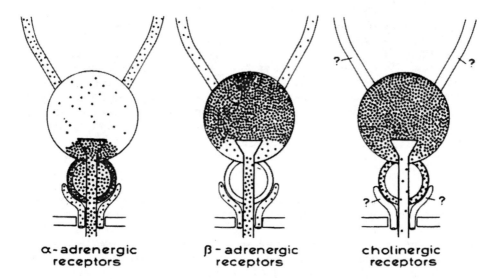

α - adrenergic   β - adrenergic   cholinergic
receptors   receptors   receptors

Fig. 1.7. Distribution of autonomic receptors in the human urinary tract. The relative densities are roughly indicated. The rhabdosphincter (see Chap. 3) is shown.

human ureter by electron microscopy (Schulman 1974), and there is good evidence for the presence of both alpha- and beta-adrenergic receptors, the former being excitatory and the latter inhibitory (Weiss et al. 1978). Whether the beta receptors are of the beta-1 or beta-2 type is not clear, and there is conflicting evidence concerning this in the case of the dog (Mayo and Halbert 1981). Whether or not cholinergic receptors are present in the ureter is still problematic. Whilst cholinergic agonists can produce a stimulatory effect on the ureter in the dog, this can be abolished by adrenalectomy (Labay et al. 1968), or by alpha-adrenergic blockade with phentolamine (Rose and Gillenwater 1974). These findings suggest that the action on the ureter may actually be due to the liberation of catecholamines from the adrenal medulla, or from cholinergic stimulation of the sympathetic ganglia, and consequent stimulation of the adrenergic receptors. On the other hand, there are reports that the stimulating effect produced by cholinergic agonists can be blocked by atropine, suggesting that muscarinic receptors are present. If the cholinergic nerve fibres do not supply cholinergic receptors, it is suggested that they may possibly be sensory in function (Schulman 1974).

Bladder and Urethra. In the lower urinary tract, the distribution of the autonomic receptors appears to be more clear-cut. The urinary bladder has an abundance of cholinergic receptors throughout the whole detrusor, and these are related to its active contraction in response to parasympathetic stimulation. Adrenergic receptors are also present throughout the whole of the detrusor, but here there is a clear differentiation between the distribution of the alpha and beta receptors, although both types can be demonstrated in all regions in the human bladder. In the body and dome of the bladder the vast majority of these receptors are beta in type, whereas in the base of the bladder and the region of the bladder neck they are predominantly alpha (Awad et al. 1974). It can thus be appreciated that owing to this differential distribution, sympathetic stimulation will increase the closure pressure at the bladder outlet and at the same time relax the dome of the bladder, whilst sympathetic inhibition will have the opposite effect.

The trigone is noteworthy in that cholinergic receptors are virtually absent (Caine et al. 1975). This difference from the rest of the bladder is presumably related to a difference in embryological origin: whereas the detrusor is derived from the endoderm, the trigone is of mesodermal origin (Tanagho et al. 1966). Alpha-adrenergic receptors are predominant, whereas beta receptors are negligible (Caine et al. 1975). The urethra has receptors of all three types, with the alpha-adrenergic receptors predominating over the beta receptors (Raz and Caine 1972), and the cholinergic receptors being of relatively minor importance (Ek et al. 1977).

Prostate. Smooth muscle constitutes a major part of the tissue in the prostate, and there is now abundant evidence of both noradrenergic (Baumgarten et al. 1968; Gosling and Thompson 1977) and cholinergic (Dunzendorfer et al. 1976; Vaalasti and Hervonen 1980) nerve supply to this tissue. Pharmacological studies of the surgical capsule and the hypertrophied tissue of prostates operated on for benign prostatic hypertrophy have shown that there are many alpha-adrenergic receptors but a negligible beta content, in both parts of the gland. It is noteworthy that cholinergic receptors are abundant in the capsule, but are virtually absent in the hyperplastic portion (Caine et al. 1975). It will be evident from the above that both adrenergic and cholinergic stimulation could be expected to increase the closure pressure along the urethra, particularly in the prostatic urethra, whereas adrenergic and to a lesser extent cholinergic blockade would have the opposite effect. Beta stimulation and blockade could be expected to have only a negligible effect in this respect.

Striated Muscle Sphincter. The external urethral sphincter is of particular interest with regard to the autonomic nervous system. It is composed of striated muscle and therefore, as would be expected, is under the nervous control of the somatic pudendal nerve. However, in addition, there is good evidence that there is an autonomic component in the nerve supply, derived from both the adrenergic and cholinergic fibres. This is a complex subject which is dealt with in greater detail in Chap. 3.

Actions of Drugs On and Via the Autonomic Nervous System

At the outset of this review of various pharmacological agents, it is desirable to recall that the emphasis in the present series of books is on the clinical practice of urology. Accordingly, emphasis will be placed throughout upon those drugs which have an action on the human urinary tract, and particularly those which have a place in urological therapeutics. Those which are of no practical importance will be dealt with only briefly, or not at all. At the same time, in the present section which deals with the drugs themselves, less emphasis will be placed upon those drugs which are already well established and widely used, while more consideration will be given to assessing those which are newer or more problematical.

Many of the drugs which produce an effect on the urinary tract do so by acting upon or modifying in some way the autonomic control described above. There are a variety of ways in which they can influence this mechanism, and not infrequently a given drug may do so in more than one way. The possible modes of action can be summarised as follows:

1) Direct action on peripheral neuroreceptors
2) Direct action on ganglionic receptors
3) Modification of receptor sensitivity
4) Alteration in the production or liberation of natural transmitter
5) Alteration in the removal of natural transmitter

In the majority of cases the resultant effects produced by these pharmacological agents on the urinary tract can be deduced logically from an understanding of their modes of action, together with a knowledge of the functions and distribution of the neuroreceptors as outlined above.

Direct Action on the Peripheral Neuroreceptors

The drugs acting on peripheral neuroreceptors are generally classified according to their predominant mode or site of action, but it must be realised that frequently they are not specific for one type of receptor alone. Thus, for example, most adrenergic agonists act on both alpha and beta receptors, although in varying proportions, and most muscarinic blockers have some action also on nicotinic receptors.

Drugs Acting on the Cholinergic Muscarinic Receptors

The greatest concentration of muscarinic receptors is in the bladder detrusor, which at the same time is the most powerful mass of smooth muscle in the urinary tract, and therefore the predominant effect of the drugs acting on these receptors is manifest by alterations in the tone and contractions of the detrusor. A minor effect is produced in the urethra and prostatic capsule.

Muscarinic Agonists. The natural neurotransmitter acetylcholine, which produces a pronounced effect in vitro, is not of use clinically because of its very rapid breakdown by acetylcholinesterase, as well as its widespread effects on other organs and systems throughout the body. In addition, its concomitant powerful action on the nicotinic receptors can produce unwanted and sometimes conflicting reactions. A number of other agents which act predominantly as muscarinic agonists, and in which the nicotinic agonist action has been greatly reduced or virtually abolished by modification of the acetylcholine molecule, are used for their actions on the urinary tract muscle. These include bethanechol chloride (Urecholine), carbachol (Doryl), and to a lesser extent methacholine (Mecholyl). These compounds are all relatively resistant to cholinesterase, the first two of them virtually not being hydrolysed at all, and the last being hydrolysed only very slowly. As a result their effects are prolonged. Their principal use is to increase the tone and contractile power of the bladder, particularly in cases of detrusor hypotonicity of various aetiologies. At the same time, by their action on the muscarinic receptors in the prostatic capsule they can increase the closure pressure in the prostatic urethra, particularly in the presence of benign prostatic hyperplasia, and hence may increase the degree of functional obstruction.

As with all such drugs, it must constantly be remembered that their effects are not confined to the urinary tract, but that they also produce effects on other organs in the body. This must be taken into account when prescribing them, and may restrict their use. Thus, for example, these muscarinic agonists may be contraindicated in asthmatic patients because of their bronchoconstricting effects, or in patients suffering from hyperthyroidism because of the possibility that they may induce atrial fibrillation.

Muscarinic Blockers. The muscarinic blockers are used mainly to diminish untoward activity and an excessive force of contraction of the bladder detrusor, particularly that seen as a result of supranuclear spinal lesions causing neurogenic bladder hyperreflexia, where the effect is usually clearly demonstrable. They are used also in a variety of other types of detrusor irritability of less clear aetiology, such as 'idiopathic' detrusor instability and enuresis nocturna, but here the response is often less definite. It is noteworthy that it has been shown experimentally that whereas they are effective blockers of parasympathomimetic drugs, they are only partially effective in blocking the muscarinic effect of parasympathetic nerve stimulation. The reason for this is obscure, but is referred to again below when considering the 'purinergic' nervous system.

The classical muscarinic blockers are atropine and the related belladonna alkaloids. However, although they are still occasionally used, their lack of specificity limits their clinical value, and the synthetic quaternary compounds such as methantheline (Banthine) and propantheline (Pro-Banthine) are much more widely used for their effects on the urinary tract. Both these drugs have some blocking effect on the nicotinic receptors in the autonomic ganglia, in addition to their predominant antimuscarinic properties. This is relatively less pronounced in the case of propantheline, which has a more potent effect on the lower urinary tract.

Emepronium bromide (Cetiprin) is another quaternary compound with both muscarinic and nicotinic blocking actions in which considerable interest has been shown in recent years, and concerning which there are conflicting reports. There seems little doubt that when given parenterally in relatively large doses it can increase bladder capacity, delay the first desire to void, and diminish the intravesical pressure in patients with uninhibited bladder detrusors (Ritch et al. 1977), although it appears to have little effect on the normal bladder (Ekeland and Sander 1976). Brocklehurst et al. (1969) have claimed it to be of particular value in relieving senile nocturnal frequency. More recently, however, Walter et al. (1982) were unable to substantiate any significant effect on urinary incontinence or uninhibited bladder contractions in a group of elderly patients when it was compared with a placebo. Similarly, Perera et al. (1982) did not find it to be of significant value in the small-capacity hyperreflexic bladders of elderly people. One of the problems arising in the case of this drug may be the poor and unreliable absorption when it is administered orally, probably not more than 2.5%–5% being absorbed. Another reason for the discrepancies reported may be variations in the exact aetiology and underlying pathology causing the bladder dysfunction in the different groups examined. At the present stage the evidence seems to indicate that it is an effective drug when given in adequate doses parenterally, but that when administered orally large doses are required and its effect is unreliable.

Diethylaminoethyl benzilate methobromide (Paragone) is a synthetic drug produced in Israel which has a similar action. It has been found to be highly effective in diminishing bladder hyperactivity (Caine 1969), and is widely used in that country for this purpose. Hyoscine butylbromide (Buscopan) is another muscarinic blocking agent, related to atropine, which is claimed to be of value in the urinary tract, particularly for the relief of ureteric colic and bladder spasms. Laval and Lutzeyer (1980) found that when administered intramuscularly it was effective in inhibiting uncontrolled detrusor contractions and increasing the bladder capacity. However, it has not found general acceptance for urological use.

In addition to the above-mentioned drugs, a number of other pharmacological agents such as oxybutynin, dicyclomine, bromocriptine and the phenothiazines show muscarinic blocking effects in addition to their main actions. They will be dealt with under their appropriate headings in the next chapter.

Drugs Acting on the Adrenergic Receptors

As indicated above there are two main groups of adrenergic receptors, with roughly opposite effects. Stimulation of the alpha receptors causes increased tone and activity of the smooth muscle, and in accordance with their distribution this effect is seen particularly in the base of the bladder, bladder neck and prostatic urethra. Stimulation of the beta receptors, on the other hand, causes relaxation of the muscle, particularly in the dome of the bladder. The blocking agents have the opposite effects.

Adrenergic Agonists. Many of the adrenergic agonists produce an effect upon both the alpha and the beta receptors, although in varying proportions. The naturally occurring neurotransmitter noradrenaline stimulates both types, with a predominant effect on the alpha receptors, but is not of any practical clinical value in relation to the urinary tract because of its widespread and powerful effects in the body, especially the cardiovascular system, and its relatively short duration of action. Adrenaline also acts on both types of receptors, but in the case of this compound beta receptors have a lower threshold of sensitivity than the alpha receptors. This can result in a diphasic type of reaction in a tissue containing both types of receptors and with a preponderance of the alpha receptors. A low concentration of adrenaline, acting on only the beta receptors, can cause relaxation whereas a higher concentration, affecting also the predominant alpha receptors, will then produce an increase in tone. Dopamine, the immediate precursor in the synthesis of noradrenaline, also has a direct stimulating action on both the alpha and the beta receptors in the vesico-urethral muscle. Although peripheral dopamine receptors are known to exist in the body, there is evidence that in this instance the effect is mediated through the adrenergic receptors themselves, rather than through any dopamine receptors.

In contrast to the above, some drugs show a great predominance of effect on one or other type of receptor. Thus phenylephrine (Neosynephrine) and methoxamine (Vasoxyl) stimulate almost exclusively the alpha receptors, whilst isoprenaline (isoproterenol; Isuprel) acts almost entirely on the beta receptors. It will be recalled that each type of adrenergic receptor can be divided into subgroups, and certain drugs have specific effects on these subgroups. For example, salbutamol and terbutaline affect principally the beta-2 receptors, and have been shown to produce a corresponding effect on the urinary tract muscle. Specific beta-1 agonists exist, such as Dobutamine, but these do not appear to influence the urinary tract, suggesting that only beta-2 receptors are present in this muscle. Clonidine has a specific stimulating effect on the alpha-2 (presynaptic) receptors, and as such the effect is of particular interest. As the action of the alpha-2 receptors is to regulate the production and liberation of noradrenaline by a negative feedback mechanism, their stimulation by clonidine will result in a decreased liberation of noradrenaline from the nerve endings. As the clonidine itself is not an agonist for the alpha-1 (postsynaptic) receptors, this means that there will be less stimulation of these receptors. The net effect of clonidine, therefore, although it is an alpha stimulator, is to produce a reduction in alpha activity, an effect that has been demonstrated on the human urethra (Nordling et al. 1979).

Adrenergic Blockers. Effective blockers exist for both the alpha and beta receptors, and they are more specific for each of these types than are the agonists. Here again, some of the blockers act on both subgroups of the receptors, whilst others are virtually specific for one subgroup.

The alpha-adrenergic blocker most widely used for its effect on the urinary tract is phenoxybenzamine (Dibenyline, Dibenzyline), which acts mainly on the alpha-1 receptors but also, especially in high concentrations, on the alpha-2 receptors. The latter effect results in an increased liberation of noradrenaline from the adrenergic nerve terminals, as explained above, which may contribute towards the tachycardia commonly produced by this drug. It is absorbed by mouth, accumulates in the body over about a week, and produces a well-maintained effect. Although it has a generalised influence on the alpha receptors throughout the body, those in the urinary tract appear to be relatively sensitive to it, and in practice it is usually possible to obtain a satisfactory response in the urinary tract with a small dose, with relatively mild side-effects on the rest of the body. As could be anticipated, the effect on the urinary tract consists in a reduction of tone in the smooth muscle of the bladder base, bladder neck, prostate and prostatic capsule, and urethra, in all of which the alpha-adrenergic receptors are predominant. Because of these effects it is widely used in order to diminish the outflow tract resistance to micturition in a variety of clinical conditions, as elaborated in subsequent chapters. It was mentioned earlier that inhibitory alpha-adrenergic receptors are present in parasympathetic ganglia, and phenoxybenzamine, by blocking these, can result in facilitation of the transmission of parasympathetic impulses (Saum and de Groat 1972). In addition, there are a number of other pharmacological effects including histamine and 5-hydroxytryptamine blockade. However, the predominant effect of phenoxybenzamine on the urinary tract remains that of alpha blockade.

Phentolamine (Regitine) is also an effective alpha-adrenergic blocker acting on both subgroups of alpha receptors. It is poorly absorbed by mouth and needs to be administered parenterally, thus resulting in a rapid but short-lived effect. As such, it can be useful when an immediate effect is required (Caine et al. 1976), or as a rapid test for assessing the likely effectiveness of other alpha blockers (Awad et al. 1976; Olsson et al. 1977). It has also been advocated for use in ureteric colic due to ureteric calculi, where it is hoped that a blocking effect on the alpha receptors in the ureter will result in inhibition of the muscle spasm and facilitate the passage of the stone (Kubacz and Catchpole 1972).

Prazosin (Minipress) is widely used as an antihypertensive drug, and acts as a selective blocker of the postsynaptic alpha-1 receptors. Because of its virtual lack of action on the presynaptic receptors it does not interfere with the regulatory feedback control of noradrenaline release, and probably for this reason produces relatively little tachycardia. It has been shown to result in a blocking effect on the alpha receptors in the human urethra (Andersson et al. 1981) and the human prostate (Shapiro et al. 1981), and may prove to be of clinical value in urological practice in the future. Yohimbine is said to be a specific blocker of the alpha-2 receptors, but is not of practical use for this purpose in urology.

In view of the clinical value of alpha-adrenergic blockers on the urinary tract, it is likely that new compounds of this type will be investigated in the future for this effect, and some of these may enter into clinical use. One of these, nicergoline, with a predominant action on the postsynaptic receptors, has already been tested experimentally by ourselves, and has been found to produce an alpha-adrenergic blocking effect on both the canine urethra and the human prostate. A report of a clinical trial of its effectiveness in the relief of benign prostatic hypertrophy has recently appeared in the literature (Ronchi et al. 1982).

In addition to the drugs used primarily for their alpha-adrenergic blocking effects, others which are used for entirely different purposes may unexpectedly produce an alpha blocking effect on the urinary tract sufficient to become manifest clinically. This was observed with diphenylhydantoin sodium (phenytoin sodium), a drug commonly used in the treatment of epilepsy. As a result of the observations that stress incontinence appeared for the first time in a number of women upon receiving this drug, appropriate investigations revealed that it produces a definite alpha-adrenergic blocking effect on the smooth muscle of the urethra, which can be sufficient to impair urethral closure in the susceptible case (Raz et al. 1973b).

Amongst the beta-adrenergic blockers, probably the best known is propranolol (Inderal, Deralin), which has a blocking effect on both the beta-1 and the beta-2 receptors. Experimentally it can be shown to produce the anticipated increased tone and activity of the detrusor (Edvardsen 1968), but this is of no practical clinical value. It can also, by virtue of blocking the beta receptors in the urethra and allowing the alpha receptors to work unopposed, increase the outflow resistance from the bladder, an action which has been of clinical use in some cases of urinary incontinence. In the case of the beta receptors also, there are drugs which have a selective blocking effect on the subgroups. Atenolol and practolol produce this action specifically on the beta-1 receptors, and butoxamine on the beta-2 receptors. As mentioned earlier, there is some evidence that the beta receptors of the urinary tract are beta-2 in nature, and therefore the specificity of blockers for the beta subgroups may prove to be of practical importance to the urologist.

Drugs Having Combined Actions

Some drugs appear to have multiple effects on the autonomic receptors, which may either reinforce each other or counteract each other. For example, isoxsuprine hydrochloride (Duvadilan) has both an alpha blocking and a beta stimulating action, the latter apparently acting predominantly on the beta-2 receptors. The combination of the two actions on the urethra would supplement each other in reducing the outflow resistance—an effect which has been found to be of some practical clinical value. Bromocriptine (Parlodel), whose primary use is for its properties as a dopamine agonist and prolactin inhibitor, has been shown to produce a blocking effect on both the alpha-adrenergic receptors and on the muscarinic cholinergic receptors, as well as to have a direct stimulating action on the human detrusor and prostatic muscle. The net resultant effect on a given tissue will, in such a case, depend on the receptors present and on the basic state of autonomic activity acting on that tissue at a given time (Ron et al. 1980; Shapiro et al. 1980). These complex actions may account for the conflicting reports that have appeared in the literature with regard to the effect of bromocriptine on the lower urinary tract in the human (Farrar and Osborne 1976; Farrar and Pryor 1976; Abrams and Dunn 1979), and taking them all into account has enabled it to be used with benefit in certain selected cases of lower urinary tract dysfunction.

Direct Action on the Ganglionic Receptors

As described previously, transmission in the autonomic ganglia is mainly due to acetylcholine liberated from the preganglionic neurons activating the nicotinic receptors of the postganglionic neurons, but it is possible that other types of transmission are also involved. Evidence exists for the presence of muscarinic receptors in the ganglia, and there is little doubt that catecholamine receptors are also present. Both alpha- and beta-adrenergic receptors can be detected, with the alpha receptors producing an inhibitory effect on ganglionic transmission and the beta receptors facilitating it. As the alpha receptors are predominant, adrenergic stimulation will normally result in the inhibition of transmission. Nevertheless, the major form of transmission is undoubtedly that of acetylcholine stimulation of the nicotinic receptors. It should be remembered that these receptors are present in both the parasympathetic and sympathetic ganglia, as well as in the adrenal medulla (which can be likened to a sympathetic ganglion), and therefore drugs affecting these receptors can result in complex effects on the body.

Ganglion Agonists

Nicotine itself has a diphasic effect on the nicotinic receptors, causing stimulation in small doses but blockade in higher doses. This blocking action may be due to persisting depolarisation of the effector cell membrane rendering it refractory to further impulses, or it may be due to a true blockade of the receptors following initial stimulation. Despite the very large amount of experimental work done with nicotine throughout the years, and the fact that it may be regarded as perhaps the most widely used drug in the world, it has no clinical application in urology. Some of the synthetic muscarinic agonists, such as bethanechol and carbachol, have a mild stimulating effect also on the nicotinic ganglionic receptors, and other more specific agonists such as tetramethylammonium (TMA) and 1,1-dimethyl-4-phenylpiperazinium iodide (DMPP) exist and are of experimental value, but none of these is of clinical importance.

Ganglion Blockers

The ganglion blockers, on the other hand, are of clinical value, although their use has declined considerably in recent years. The quaternary ammonium compounds such as methantheline, propantheline and emepronium, as mentioned earlier, have nicotinic blocking effects as well as their muscarinic blocking actions. However, other compounds such as tetraethylammonium (TEA) and hexamethonium, or the newer drugs such as pentolinium (Ansolysin), mecamylamine (Inversine) and trimetaphan camsylate (Arfonad) all have a pronounced and specific blocking action on the nicotinic receptors. Their main clinical use has been for their actions on sympathetic ganglionic transmission and the resultant effects on the cardiovascular system, particularly for the treatment of hypertension. However, because of their concomitant actions on the parasympathetic ganglia, they can affect the functions of the bladder detrusor, and may cause difficulty in micturition or even complete retention of urine. In addition, they may cause interference with erection due to blockade of the parasympathetic transmission to the nervi erigentes, and abolish ejaculation due to blockade of the sympathetic transmission to the vasa deferentia, seminal vesicles and prostate.

The ganglion blockers are of use in urological practice for the treatment of autonomic dysreflexia (autonomic hyperreflexia). This condition, seen in spinal cord lesions above the level of thoracic segment 5, is due to widespread over-activity involving both the sympathetic and parasympathetic systems caused by lack of normal control of the spinal autonomic reflexes, as a result of interruption of the spinal pathways normally subserving this control. As a result, afferent stimuli reaching the spinal cord below the level of the lesion cause an excessive sympathetic discharge with an associated liberation of noradrenaline, the metabolites of which can be shown to increase in the urine. This excessive sympathetic activity results in marked vasoconstriction, particularly of the splanchnic vascular bed, resulting in severe hypertension. This in turn acts on the baroreceptors in the aortic arch and on the carotid sinus, causing vagal stimulation and bradycardia. From the account of this mechanism, it can be appreciated that one of the modes of treatment would logically be to interrupt the transmission at the autonomic ganglia, and both pentolinium in repeated subcutaneous doses of 2 mg, and trimetaphan camsylate by slow intravenous infusion at a concentration of 1 mg/ml, have been found to be effective treatments for this condition. The subject of autonomic dysreflexia is considered further in Chap. 5.

Modification of Receptor Sensitivity

It was mentioned earlier that the autonomic receptors are not fixed, immutable entities, but that their nature or sensitivity can be altered by various factors. These may be physical factors such as variations in temperature, alterations in muscle tension, or the presence of obstruction in the case of the bladder detrusor, or they may be hormonal factors. The changes in autonomic receptor response due to variations in the female sex hormone milieu have been well recognised for many years in the case of the uterine muscle, but more recently it has become evident that female sex hormones can also cause comparable changes in the muscle of the urinary tract.

Our studies have indicated that an increase in the level of oestrogens can increase the sensitivity of the alpha-adrenergic receptors, whereas an increase in the level of progestogens can increase the sensitivity of the beta-adrenergic receptors (Caine and Raz 1975). In the rabbit, administration of oestrogens has been found to increase the response of the bladder and urethra to alpha-adrenergic stimulation (Hodgson et al. 1978). More recently, Levin et al. (1981) have produced evidence that in the rabbit detrusor, oestrogen administration increases the density of both the alpha-adrenergic receptors and the cholinergic muscarinic receptors, and causes a marked increase in the contractile response to both alpha-adrenergic and cholinergic stimulation. No effect was noted on the beta-adrenergic response or receptor density.

These observations can be of clinical importance both in relation to the variations in hormone levels that occur naturally in women during the menstrual cycle, pregnancy and the menopause, and in relation to the effects on the urinary tract produced by administration of the hormones. In the former instance, the increase in sensitivity of the beta receptors as the result of increased progesterone levels may be one of the causal factors for the ureteric dilatation seen in pregnancy (Raz et al. 1972b). It may also explain the worsening of mild incontinence often encountered during pregnancy, and the variation in the degree of incontinence seen in the different phases of the menstrual cycle. The latter correlates well with the increased closure pressure in the urethra during the oestrogen phase of the menstrual cycle, and the decrease in closure pressure in the progesterone phase, found by Schreiter et al. (1976).

It is well recognised that oestrogen administration can be of benefit in the treatment of mild cases of stress incontinence, especially in post-menopausal women. In this instance the oestrogens probably produce their effects by a variety of mechanisms. They act on the oestrogen-sensitive urethral mucosa, improving its thickness and elasticity; they cause proliferation and engorgement of the submucosal vascular channels, which contribute nearly a third to the effective closure of the urethra (Raz et al. 1972a); and in addition they increase the sensitivity of the alpha-adrenergic receptors in the urethral and bladder neck muscle to the local and circulating catecholamines, resulting in an increased muscular tone and an improved closure pressure at these sites (Raz et al. 1973c). Conversely, because of their facilitating effects on the beta-adrenergic receptors, the progestogens can have the opposite effect on the urethra. We have shown experimentally that administration of progesterone will result in a change in the response of the canine urethra to noradrenaline from an alpha-mediated contraction to a beta-mediated relaxation (Raz et al. 1973a). Clinically, we found that administration of medroxyprogesterone acetate to women with mild stress incontinence considerably worsened the condition in 60% of the cases, at the same time diminishing the urethral closure pressure. This effect passed off after cessation of the treatment (Raz et al. 1973c). This effect of progestogens on the urethral beta receptors may also occur in the male, and this possibility must be taken into account when assessing any effects apparently produced by this type of hormonal treatment given for benign prostatic hyperplasia.

Alteration in the Production or Liberation of Natural Transmitter

It is clear that one of the ways in which drugs could produce an autonomic effect would be by altering the production or liberation of the natural neurotransmitter rather than, or in addition to, themselves having a direct effect on the receptors. A number of drugs acting in this manner on the synthesis of noradrenaline are of relevance to the urinary tract.

As outlined above, noradrenaline is produced in the sympathetic neurons from tyrosine, via the intermediate stages of levodopa and dopamine, and normally the rate-limiting stage in this biosynthesis is the step from tyrosine to levodopa, catalysed by tyrosine hydroxylase. Administration of levodopa by-passes this step, resulting in an increased production of dopamine and noradrenaline. In addition to this, levodopa apparently displaces the noradrenaline from the peripheral sympathetic nerve endings (Liu et al. 1971). Although the drug itself does not appear to have any direct effect on the vesico-urethral musculature in vitro, it does produce an adrenergic effect in vivo, presumably due to the above mechanism (Benson et al. 1976). This presumably accounts for the bladder outlet obstruction and difficulty in micturition experienced by some patients receiving levodopa treatment for parkinsonism (Murdoch et al. 1975).

Ephedrine, its stereo-isomer pseudoephedrine (Sudafed), and phenylpropan-olamine (contained in Ornade spansules) produce liberation of noradrenaline from the neuronal vesicles, as well as having a direct agonistic effect on both the alpha and beta receptors. They are all active when taken by mouth, and have been shown to increase the urethral closure pressure in the human. Because of its effect on the urethra, ephedrine has been used to improve continence both in patients suffering from stress incontinence and in those suffering from post-prostatectomy incontinence. Diokno and Taub (1975), using dosages of up to 200 mg a day, obtained good results in 27 out of 38 patients and were able to demonstrate an improved closure on the urethral pressure profile recording. Khanna (1976) obtained a similar result using from 50 to 100 mg a day. This adrenergic effect on the prostatic smooth muscle in the patient with an enlarged prostate can increase the micturition difficulty and even result in acute retention of urine, a complication of ephedrine therapy recognised as long ago as 1928 by Boston. Ephedrine therapy is characterised by the frequent appearance of tachyphylaxis, possibly because of depletion of the noradrenaline stores. Side-effects including anxiety and nervousness, insomnia and tachycardia are not uncommon, and its action on the blood vessels results in a rise in blood pressure, which limits its use in hypertensive patients. Phenylpropanolamine in the form of Ornade spansules has also been found to benefit some patients with stress incontinence and post-prostatectomy incontinence (Stewart et al. 1976), and has the advantage of producing less central stimulating effect than ephedrine.

Guanethidine (Ismelin) and bretylium (Bretylate) have an opposite type of action, preventing liberation of noradrenaline from the neuronal vesicles into the synaptic cleft. They are of no practical use in the urinary tract, but have been reported to produce sphincter incompetence and loss of ejaculation when used for the treatment of hypertension (Boura and Green 1965). Reserpine depletes the intraneuronal stores, apparently by causing release of noradrena-line and preventing its reaccumulation. Its use for hypertension has been reported to cause stress incontinence in women (Kleeman 1970). Methyldopa (Aldomet) is closely related to levodopa, and interferes with the synthesis of noradrenaline by competing for the enzyme levodopa decarboxylase which converts the levodopa into dopamine. This results in the production of a relati-vely inactive 'false transmitter' methylnoradrenaline, instead of the normal noradrenaline. Clinical evidence of a reduction in sympathetic stimulation of the lower urinary tract has been observed in patients taking this drug for the treatment of hypertension, and Raz (1974) reported a case in which stress incontinence associated with a reduction in the urethral pressure profile was associated with this treatment. Out of a series of 38 patients with neurogenic bladder dysfunction of the upper motor neuron type, improvement was obtained with methyldopa treatment in 29 (Raz et al. 1977). In this instance, however, an objective effect on the urethral pressure profile was not so marked, and it was postulated that the effect might be due to a central action rather than a peripheral one.

Alteration in the Removal of Natural Transmitter

Normally, the natural transmitters are deactivated or removed very rapidly from the site of their action, and it is evident that interference with this normal process would result in a prolongation and intensification of the action of the transmitter involved.

In the case of acetylcholine, as already described, deactivation is produced locally by acetylcholinesterase, and a number of drugs are in use which can inactivate this enzyme. Physostigmine (eserine) was probably the first of these agents to be used, and is well absorbed by mouth, but its main use at the present time is for its local effect in the form of eye drops. Neostigmine (Prostigmin) is poorly absorbed by mouth and, as its effects at the nicotinic receptor sites of striated muscle are predominant, it is mainly used to counteract the effects of the d-tubocurarine type of drugs on the neuromuscular junction, and in the treatment of myasthaenia gravis. Both drugs can be shown to have an effect on the bladder detrusor, increasing its response to cholinergic stimulation, the effect of neostigmine being more prolonged than that of physostigmine. It has been used for the treatment of post-operative urinary retention, but is rarely used for this purpose nowadays.

Intrathecal injections of neostigmine have also been used in order to produce erection and ejaculation in paraplegic patients (Guttmann and Walsh 1971). Doses of the order of 0.25–0.30 mg of neostigmine methyl sulphate are used, and in successful cases erection and ejaculation usually occur about 1–3 hours later. The erection usually persists for a considerable time, and the ejaculations are often repeated several times during the period of erection. This method has been used in order to obtain semen for artificial insemination in the wives of paraplegic patients who fail to get ejaculation during intercourse (Spira 1956).

A newer anticholinesterase, distigmine bromide (Ubretid), has a similar but more prolonged action to that of neostigmine, and has been recommended for its cholinergic action on the urinary bladder, both for post-operative retention and for neurogenic bladders, but only those of the upper motor neuron type (Yeo et al. 1974). Although it is relatively poorly absorbed from the gastro-intestinal tract it is effective in doses of 5 mg orally, as well as intramuscularly in doses of 0.5 mg.

Neuronally liberated noradrenaline is mainly inactivated by re-uptake into the adrenergic neurons, and therefore prevention of this uptake would logically increase its effect. Imipramine (Tofranil) is reputed to have a number of modes of action on the urinary tract, one of the main ones apparently being to block this re-uptake of noradrenaline. Experimental evidence for this effect on the urinary tract in the dog was found by Khanna et al. (1975), who demonstrated that administration of imipramine produced an increased urethral pressure which could be blocked by phenoxybenzamine. Mahoney et al. (1973) found a similar effect on the urethral closure pressure in children treated for urinary incontinence. Conflicting opinions exist as to whether or not imipramine has in addition a muscarinic blocking effect on the detrusor. A blocking effect on acetylcholine-induced contractions of muscle strips taken from dog and rabbit detrusors has been described (Labay and Boyarsky 1973), and an inhibiting action on the bladder contractions caused by pelvic nerve stimulation in dogs, comparable to that obtained with propantheline, was reported by Gregory et al. (1974). On the other hand, Diokno et al. (1972) found no demonstrable anticholinergic effect of imipramine on the uncontrolled contractions of the uninhibited neurogenic bladder, even with parenteral doses as high as 75 mg, whereas propantheline had a pronounced muscarinic blocking effect on these contractions. It may be that these conflicting results are explained to some extent by species differences, and that even if a muscarinic blocking action on the bladder detrusor in man does exist, it is so weak as to be of no practical significance. In addition to these two types of action, imipramine undoubtedly has a central effect which may reflect on the urinary tract function, and there is good evidence also for a direct relaxant effect on the muscle itself (see Chap. 2).

Nortriptyline (Aventyl) is another tricyclic antidepressant which is closely related to imipramine, and has been shown to produce a similar beneficial effect on the lower urinary tract in man, both in cases of enuresis (Litvak et al. 1968) and in patients with irritative bladder symptoms (Servadio et al. 1975).

Purinergic and Peptidergic Nerves

Purinergic Nerves

It has been known for many years that the parasympathetic vagal supply to the stomach includes inhibitory as well as stimulatory fibres, and that these fibres are not adrenergic in nature. Similarly, it is known that whereas atropine can effectively block the muscarinic cholinergic receptors in the bladder, it is only incompletely effective in blocking the stimulatory effects of pelvic nerve stimulation on the bladder. These observations have led to the suggestion that in addition to the sympathetic and parasympathetic pathways there exists another nervous pathway that travels together with the parasympathetic nerves, but in which the neurotransmitter is not acetylcholine but possibly an adenine nucleotide, either adenosine triphosphate (ATP) or a closely related compound (Burnstock et al. 1972).

Intra-arterial injection of ATP close to the bladder in the dog can produce a response corresponding to about 50% of that produced by nerve stimulation. However, although quinidine, which blocks the effects of ATP on intestinal muscle, produced some reduction in the bladder response to nerve stimulation, it did not have this effect on the injected ATP (Creed and Tulloch 1978). There is experimental evidence that the detrusor contraction produced by ATP may in part be mediated by prostaglandins (see Chap. 2) released locally by the ATP, and that both ATP and prostaglandins may contribute to the non-adrenergic, non-cholinergic component of bladder contraction (Andersson et al. 1980).

The existence of purinergic nerve fibres is not accepted by all authorities, and critics suggest that the observed reactions may be explained by other mechanisms, such as antidromal impulses passing in a reverse direction along sensory nerves, or substances produced locally as the result of the experimental electrical stimulation. At present the issue is undecided, and does not appear to be of practical pharmacological importance.

Peptidergic Nerves

There is increasing evidence that various peptides may be produced by certain neurons and act as neurotransmitters, and some of these may ultimately prove to be of importance in the urinary tract. Possibly the most widely distributed of these is that known as the Vasoactive Intestinal Polypeptide (VIP), which is a potent vasodilator and a relaxer of non-vascular smooth muscle. It has been shown to have an inhibitory effect on the rabbit bladder detrusor in vitro, an action which is not blocked by propranolol, and shows no difference in reaction between the body and the base of the bladder (Levin and Wein 1981). Nerves containing VIP have been demonstrated in both the cat prostate (Larsson et al. 1977; Alm et al. 1977) and the human prostate (Vaalasti et al. 1980), as well as in the ureter. Its action is dependent on calcium ions, is not blocked by atropine, and has no known specific blockers.

Every clinician is well aware that the treatment of bladder dysfunction of the hyperactive type with muscarinic blockers is often relatively ineffective, and the results disappointing. In view of the above findings, the possibility arises that the parasympathetic non-cholinergic nerves may play a role in bladder contractility, and may be of functional significance in this type of case. Although the pharmacological manipulation of the purinergic and peptidergic nerves is not, at the time of writing, of practical clinical application, it may well prove to be so in the future, and hence the above very brief review of the subject is included.

References

Abrams PH, Dunn M (1979) A double blind trial of bromocriptine in the treatment of idiopathic bladder instability. Br J Urol 51:24–27

Ahlquist RP (1948) A study of adrenotropic receptors. Am J Physiol 153:586–600

Alm P, Alumets J, Håkanson R, Sundler F (1977) Peptidergic (vasoactive intestinal peptide) nerves in the genito-urinary tract. Neuroscience 2:751–754

Andersson K-E, Husted S, Sjögren C (1980) Contribution of prostaglandins to the adenosine triphosphate-induced contraction of rabbit urinary bladder. Br J Pharmacol 70:443–452

Andersson K-E, Ek A, Hedlund H, Mattiasson A (1981) Effects of prazosin on isolated human urethra and in patients with lower motor neuron lesions. Invest Urol 19:39–42

Awad SA, Bruce AW, Carro-Ciampi G, Downie JW, Lin M (1974) Distribution of α and β adrenoceptors in human urinary bladder. Br J Pharmacol 50:525–529

Awad SA, Downie JW, Lywood DW, Young RA, Jarzylo SV (1976) Sympathetic activity in the proximal urethra in patients with urinary obstruction. J Urol 115:545–547

Baumgarten HG, Falck B, Holstein AF, Owman Ch, Owman T (1968) Adrenergic innervation of the human testis, epididymis, ductus deferens and prostate: A fluorescence microscopic and fluorimetric study. Z Zellforsch mikrosk Anat 90:81–95

Belleau B (1963) An analysis of drug receptor interactions. In: Modern concepts in the relationship between structure and pharmacological activity. Proceedings of the First International Pharmacological Meeting 1961, vol 7. Pergamon Press, London, pp 75–99

Benson GS, Raezer DM, Anderson JR, Saunders CD, Corriere JN (1976). Effect of levodopa on urinary bladder. Urology 7:24–28

Berthelsen S, Pettinger WA (1977) A functional basis for classification of α-adrenergic receptors. Life Sci 21:595

Boston LN (1928) Dysuria following ephedrine therapy. Med Rec 56:94–95

Boura ALA, Green AF (1965) Adrenergic neurone blocking agents. Annu Rev Pharmacol 5:183–212

Brocklehurst JC, Dillane JB, Fry J, Armitage P (1969) Clinical trial of emepronium bromide in nocturnal frequency of old age. Br Med J 2:216–218

Burnstock G, Dumsday B, Smythe A (1972) Atropine resistant excitation of the urinary bladder: the possibility of transmission via nerve releasing a purine nucleotide. Br J Pharmacol 44:451–461

Caine M (1969) The effect of Paragone on the human bladder. Israel J Med Sci 5:1037–1043

Caine M, Raz S (1975) Some clinical implications of adrenergic receptors in the urinary tract. Arch Surg 110:247–250

Caine M, Raz S, Zeigler M (1975) Adrenergic and cholinergic receptors in the human prostate, prostatic capsule and bladder neck. Br J Urol 47:193–202

Caine M, Pfau A, Perlberg S (1976) The use of alpha-adrenergic blockers in benign prostatic obstruction. Br J Urol 48:255–263

Creed KE, Tulloch AGS (1978) The effect of pelvic nerve stimulation and some drugs on the urethra and bladder of the dog. Br J Urol 50:398–405

de Groat WC, Saum WR (1971) Adrenergic inhibition in mammalian parasympathetic ganglia. Nature [New Biol] 231:188–189

Diokno AC, Taub M (1975) Ephedrine in treatment of urinary incontinence. Urology 5:624–625

Diokno AC, Hyndman CW, Hardy DA, Lapides J (1972) Comparison of action of imipramine (Tofranil) and propantheline (Probanthine) on detrusor contraction. J Urol 107:42–43

Dunzendorfer U, Jonas D, Weber W (1976) The autonomic innervation of the human prostate. Histochemistry of acetylcholinesterase in the normal and pathologic states. Urol Res 4:29–31

Edvardsen P (1968) Nervous control of urinary bladder in cats. III. Effects of autonomic blocking agents in the intact animal. Acta Physiol Scand 72:183–193

Ek A, Alm P, Andersson K-E, Persson CGA (1977) Adrenoceptor and cholinoceptor mediated responses of the isolated human urethra. Scand J Urol Nephrol 11:97–102

Ekeland A, Sander S (1976) A urodynamic study of emepronium bromide in bladder dysfunction. Scand J Urol Nephrol 10:195–199

Elbadawi A, Schenk EA (1971) A new theory of the innervation of bladder musculature. 3. Postganglionic synapses in uretero-vesico-urethral autonomic pathways. J Urol 105:372–374

Farrar DJ, Osborne JL (1976) The use of bromocriptine in the treatment of the unstable bladder. Br J Urol 48:235–238

Farrar DJ, Pryor JS (1976) The effect of bromocriptine in patients with benign prostatic hypertrophy. Br J Urol 48:73–75

Gosling JA, Thompson SA (1977) A neurohistochemical and histological study of peripheral autonomic neurons of the human bladder neck and prostate. Urol Int 32:269–276

Gregory JG, Wein AJ, Schoenberg HW (1974) A comparison of the action of Tofranil and Probanthine on the urinary bladder. Invest Urol 12:233–235

Guttmann L, Walsh JJ (1971) Prostigmin assessment test of fertility in spinal man. Paraplegia 9:39–51

Hodgson BJ, Dumas S, Bolling DR, Heesch CM (1978) Effect of estrogen on sensitivity of rabbit bladder and urethra to phenylephrine. Invest Urol 16:67–69

Iversen LL (1965) The uptake of catecholamines at high perfusion concentrations in the rat isolated heart: a novel catecholamine uptake process. Br J Pharmacol 25:18–33

Khanna OP (1976) Disorders of micturition: neuropharmacologic basis and results of drug therapy. Urology 8:316–328

Khanna OP, Elkouss G, Heber D, Gonick P (1975) Imipramine hydrochloride: pharmacodynamic effects on lower urinary tract of female dogs. Urology 6:48–51

Khanna OP, Barbieri EJ, McMichael RF (1981) The effects of adrenergic agonists and antagonists on vesicourethral smooth muscle of rabbit. J Pharmacol Exp Ther 216:95–100

Kleeman FJ (1970) The physiology of the internal urinary sphincter. J Urol 104:549–554

Kubacz GJ, Catchpole BN (1972) The role of adrenergic blockade in the treatment of ureteral colic. J Urol 107:949–951

Kunos G, Nickerson M (1976) Temperature-induced interconversion of α- and β-adrenoreceptors in the frog heart. J Physiol (Lond) 256:23–40

Labay P, Boyarsky S (1973) The action of imipramine on the bladder musculature. J Urol 109:385–387

Labay PC, Boyarsky S, Herlong JH (1968) Relation of adrenal to ureteral function. Fed Proc 27:444

Lands AM, Arnold A, McAuliff JP, Luduena FP, Brown TG Jr (1967) Differentiation of receptor systems activated by sympathomimetic amines. Nature 214:597–598

Larsson L-I, Fahrenkrug J, Schaffalitzky de Muckadell OB (1977) Occurrence of nerves containing vasoactive intestinal polypeptide immunoreactivity in the male genital tract. Life Sci 21:503–508

Laval K-U, Lutzeyer W (1980) Spontaneous phasic activity of the detrusor: a cause of uninhibited contractions in unstable bladders. Urol Int 35:182–187

Levin RM, Wein AJ (1981) Effect of vasoactive intestinal peptide on the contractility of the rabbit urinary bladder. Urol Res 9:217–218

Levin RM, Jacobowitz D, Wein AJ (1981) Autonomic innervation of rabbit urinary bladder following estrogen administration. Urology 17:449–453

Litvak AS, Rea M, Baker J (1968) The use of nortriptyline hydrochloride in urology. J Urol 99:462–465

Liu PL, Krenis LJ, Ngai SH (1971) The effect of levodopa on the norepinephrine stores in rat heart. Anesthesiology 34:4–8

Mahoney DT, Laferte RO, Mahoney JE (1973) Observations on sphincter-augmenting effect of imipramine in children with urinary incontinence. Urology 1:317–323

Marshall JM, Kroeger EA (1973) Adrenergic influences on uterine smooth muscle. Philos Trans R Soc Lond [Biol] 265:135–148

Mayo ME, Halbert SA (1981) The effect of autonomic drugs on ureteric peristalsis: a canine in-vivo study. Urol Res 9:209–216

Murdock MI, Olsson CA, Sax DS, Krane RJ (1975) Effect of levodopa on the bladder outlet. J Urol 113:803–805

Nordling J, Meyhoff HH, Christensen NJ (1979) Effects of clonidine (Catapresan) on urethral pressure. Invest Urol 16:289–291

Olsson CA, Siroky MB, Krane RJ (1977) The phentolamine test in neurogenic bladder dysfunction. J Urol 117:481–485

Perera GLS, Ritch AES, Hall MRP (1982) The lack of effect of intramuscular empronium bromide for urinary incontinence. Br J Urol 54:259–260

Raz S (1974) Adrenergic influence on the internal urinary sphincter. Isr J Med Sci 10:608–611

Raz S, Caine M (1972) Adrenergic receptors in the female canine urethra. Invest Urol 9:319–323

Raz S, Caine M, Zeigler M (1972a) The vascular component in the production of intraurethral pressure. J Urol 108:93–96

Raz S, Zeigler M, Caine M (1972b) Hormonal influence on the adrenergic receptors of the ureter. Br J Urol 44:405–410

Raz S, Zeigler M, Caine M (1973a) The effect of progesterone on the adrenergic receptors of the urethra. Br J Urol 45:131–135

Raz S, Zeigler M, Caine M (1973b) The effect of diphenylhydantoin on the urethra. Invest Urol 10:293–294

Raz S, Zeigler M, Caine M (1973c) The role of female hormones in stress incontinence. In: Proceedings of the 16th Congress of the International Society of Urology, vol 2. Doin, Paris, pp 397–402

Raz S, Kaufman JJ, Ellison GW, Mayers LW (1977) Methyldopa in treatment of neurogenic bladder disorders. Urology 9:188–190

Ritch AES, Castleden CM, George CF, Hall MRP (1977) A second look at emepronium bromide in urinary incontinence. Lancet I:504–506

Rohner TJ Jr, Hannigan JD, Sanford EJ (1978) Altered in-vitro adrenergic responses of dog detrusor muscle after chronic bladder outlet obstruction. Urology 11:357–361

Ron M, Shapiro A, Caine M (1980) The action of bromocriptine on human detrusor muscle. Urol Res 8:207–210

Ronchi F, Margonato A, Ceccardi R, Rigatti P, Rossini BM (1982) Symptomatic treatment of benign prostatic obstruction with nicergoline: a placebo controlled clinical study and urodynamic evaluation. Urol Res 10:131–134

Rose JG, Gillenwater JY (1974) The effect of adrenergic and cholinergic agents and their blockers upon ureteral activity. Invest Urol 11:439–451

Saum WR, de Groat WC (1972) Parasympathetic ganglia: activation of an adrenergic inhibitory mechanism by cholinomimetic agents. Science 175:659–661

Schreiter F, Fuchs P, Stockamp K (1976) Estrogenic sensitivity of alpha-receptors in the urethral musculature. Urol Int 31:13–19

Schulman CC (1974) Electron microscopy of the human ureteric innervation. Br J Urol 46:609–623

Servadio C, Nissenkorn I, Zeigler M (1975) Nortriptyline hydrochloride in urology. Urology 5:747–750

Shapiro A, Ron M, Caine M, Kramer J (1980) The pharmacological action of bromocriptine on the human prostate. Urol Res 8:25–28

Shapiro A, Mazouz B, Caine M (1981) The alpha-adrenergic blocking effect of prazosin on the human prostate. Urol Res 9:17–20

Spira R (1956) Artificial insemination after intrathecal injection of neostigmine in a paraplegic. Lancet I:670–671

Stewart BH, Banowsky LHW, Montague DK (1976) Stress incontinence: conservative therapy with sympathomimetic drugs. J Urol 115:558–559

Tanagho EA, Miller ER, Meyers FH, Corbett RK (1966) Observations on the dynamics of the bladder neck. Br J Urol 38:72–84

Vaalasti A, Hervonen A (1980) Autonomic innervation of the human prostate. Invest Urol 17:293–297

Vaalasti A, Linnoila 1, Hervonen A (1980) Immunohistochemical demonstration of VIP and enkephalin immunoreactive nerve fibres in the human prostate and seminal vesicles. Histochemistry 66:89–98

Walter S, Hansen J, Hansen L, Maegaard E, Meyhoff HH, Nordling J (1982) Urinary incontinence in old age. A controlled clinical trial of emepronium bromide. Br J Urol 54:249–251

Weiss RM, Bassett AL, Hoffman BF (1978) Adrenergic innervation of the ureter. Invest Urol 16:123–127

Yeo J, Southwell P, Rutowski S, Marchant-Williams H (1974) A further report on the effect of distigmine bromide (Ubretid) on the neurogenic bladder. Med J Aust 2:201–203

Chapter 2

Non-autonomic Drugs Acting on the Urinary Tract

Marco Caine

Direct-Acting Drugs

In addition to the drugs which produce their effects on the urinary tract musculature on or via the autonomic nervous system, there are others whose action appears to be predominantly or entirely a direct one on the muscle cell itself. The exact mechanism of this action is in most cases still obscure, and may well differ from case to case, but it is apparently not via specific receptors, nor via any neural pathway. These pharmacological agents may produce either an increase or a decrease in tone, and in the urinary tract their effects are usually manifest clinically mainly on the largest mass of smooth muscle, namely the bladder detrusor.

Stimulants

Those drugs which have a direct stimulatory action on smooth muscle are not usually employed clinically for this purpose in the urinary tract. They include such substances as ergot and some of it derivatives, digitalis glycosides, oxytocin and angiotensin. The last of these, which can be shown to produce a definite effect on the lower urinary tract muscle experimentally, is usually believed to owe this action entirely to its direct effect. However, there is now evidence that part of its action may be produced by stimulation of the alpha-adrenergic receptors, and we have found that alpha-adrenergic blocking agents can reduce the muscular response by about 50% in the experimental animal (Raz et al. 1972).

Relaxants

A number of drugs, sometimes referred to as 'musculotropic relaxants', act directly on the smooth muscle cell to produce a relaxing effect. Their site of action appears to be beyond the receptor sites on the cell membrane, and although the exact molecular mechanism is uncertain, there is evidence that at least some of the drugs, such as papaverine and flavoxate, may act by inhibiting the phosphodiesterase activity in the cell. This enzyme is normally the major agent responsible for the intracellular breakdown of cyclic AMP, and thus its inhibition would logically result in an accumulation of intracellular cyclic AMP. This in turn, as explained previously in relation to the mechanism of beta-adrenergic activation, would bring about an increased uptake of calcium ions into the intracellular stores, a reduction of free calcium ions in the sarcoplasm, and hence a decreased activity of the contractile mechanism of the smooth muscle cell (Fig. 2.1). It will be appreciated that according to these theories,

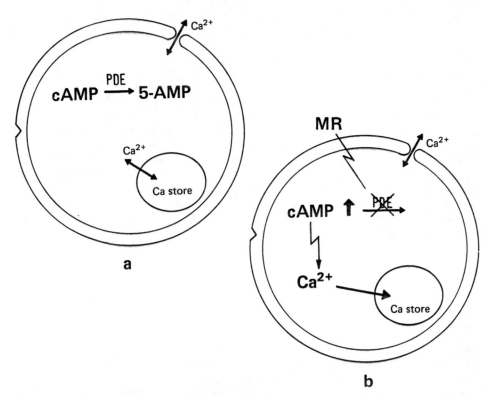

Fig. 2.1. a Normal condition in muscle cell, showing breakdown of cyclic AMP (cAMP) to 5-AMP by means of phosphodiesterase (PDE). **b** Musculotropic agent (MR) inhibits the action of phosphodiesterase (PDE), causing accumulation of cyclic AMP (cAMP) in the cell. This results in increased uptake of calcium ions (Ca^{2+}) into intracellular stores.

in both the present case and in the case of beta-adrenergic stimulation, the muscle relaxation is due to increased intracellular cyclic AMP; but whereas in the case of beta-adrenergic activity the increased cyclic AMP is the result of increased production, in the present case it is due to reduced breakdown (cf. Fig. 1.6, p.12).

A number of direct-acting smooth muscle relaxants are in clinical use for various non-urological conditions, and are of little or no practical importance from the urological point of view. Occasionally, however, concomitant effects on the urinary tract muscle may be sufficiently pronounced to become manifest clinically. Thus, for example, hydrallazine (Apresoline) produces its major action on the cardiovascular system mainly by a direct relaxing effect on the vascular muscle, and is used for the treatment of hypertension. However, a mild relaxing effect on the detrusor can also occur, and its use has led to difficulty in micturition and even retention of urine in some patients.

Papaverine is a non-specific smooth muscle relaxant used mainly for its vascular actions, whose mechanism of action is probably as described above. There are conflicting reports as to its effectiveness in the urinary tract, particularly with regard to the ureter. There seems to be some evidence that its action is more pronounced on muscle which is in spasm, and despite the lack of convincing objective evidence as to its efficacy it is still commonly used, either alone or in combination with an analgesic, for the relief of ureteric colic.

There are at present three drugs of the musculotropic relaxant type which are in common use specifically for their effects on the lower urinary tract, namely flavoxate, dicyclomine and oxybutynin. Although their main action is the direct one on the muscle, and they are accordingly classified under this heading, they all have in addition some degree of muscarinic blocking action, as well as local anaesthetic and analgesic properties.

Flavoxate hydrochloride (Urispas) has been shown to produce a significant relaxing effect, comparable to that produced by propantheline, in both normal and neurogenic bladders. Although it does possess some antimuscarinic action this is very slight, and thus the anticholinergic side-effects are very much less than those that are seen with propantheline (Kohler and Morales 1968; Bradley and Cazort 1970). In his investigation of a group of women suffering from irritative bladder symptoms such as frequency and urgency, Stanton (1973) found that flavoxate had a definite effect on the detrusor resulting in a reduced intravesical pressure, an increased vesical capacity and a delayed desire to void, accompanied by a reduction in the irritative symptoms. It did not produce any significant increase in the residual urine. In general it was found to be more effective, both in affording symptomatic relief and in producing objective cystometrographic improvement, than was emepronium bromide, with which it was compared. In addition to its relaxant properties, it also has a local anaesthetic and analgesic effect on the bladder (Setnikar et al. 1960).

Dicyclomine hydrochloride (Bentyl) also has mainly a direct action together with some antimuscarinic action, and has been shown to be capable of inhibiting detrusor contractions induced both directly and by muscarinic receptor stimulation in the experimental animal (Johns et al. 1976), as well as relaxing contraction of the urethral musculature (Khanna et al. 1979). Clinically, it can relieve irritative bladder symptoms and increase bladder capacity (Fischer et al. 1978), but it is important to note that it may take up to 10 days to produce an effect when administered orally (Awad et al. 1977).

Oxybutynin (Ditropan) has a similar dual action on the detrusor which is demonstrable both experimentally (Fredericks et al. 1975) and clinically (Diokno and Lapides 1972; Thompson and Lauvetz 1976; Moisey et al. 1980). In addition it has a local anaesthetic action, which may potentiate its antispasmodic effect. It has been reported as being effective in cases of idiopathic detrusor instability in which all other drugs had failed (Paulson 1979), and in relieving bladder spasms due to indwelling catheters and in patients after prostatectomy (Paulson 1978).

Imipramine (Tofranil) has already been referred to in the previous chapter with regard to what is probably its main mode of action in the urinary tract, namely that of interfering with the re-uptake of noradrenaline by the noradrenergic nerves, thus resulting in an increased adrenergic effect. There are probably a number of other modes of action attributable to this drug, including direct muscle relaxation and an antimuscarinic action, in addition to its antidepressant actions on the central nervous system. The question as to its antimuscarinic action and the conflicting reports concerning this, has been dealt with in Chap. 1. That the musculotropic relaxant effect is appreciable is suggested by comparative studies such as those published by Benson et al. (1977) and Fredericks et al. (1978), in which this effect was found to be comparable to that of oxybutynin and very much greater than that of flavoxate. In both these experimental studies, one on canine detrusor and the other on rabbit detrusor, flavoxate appeared to have disappointingly little effect, a finding much at variance with the results obtained in clinical practice. Such discrepancies may be explained by a variety of factors, as for example species differences or the nature of the experimental protocol. In the latter respect, barium chloride was used as a direct muscle stimulant in both the above studies, and it could well be that the postulated mode of action of flavoxate as described earlier in this chapter may be effective in a cell undergoing normal metabolism and physiological contraction, but not in one stimulated artificially by barium chloride. It serves as a reminder of the care that must always be taken in extrapolating results obtained in experimental animals to the clinical situation in human beings.

From the practical point of view, the decision as to whether to employ a muscarinic blocker or a musculotropic relaxant in a given patient, and if the latter which particular musculotropic agent to choose, is at the present time to a large extent empirical. There does not appear clinically to be a specific drug preference in a particular condition or particular type of patient (except that in patients with a hyperfunction of neuropathic origin it would appear logical to try a muscarinic blocker first), and the response seems to be largely individual. In many cases the best policy at present appears to be to assess the individual patient's response to the different drugs available, and to choose the most effective one in the given case.

Prostaglandins

The prostaglandins are a group of lipid-soluble fatty acids which were first detected in the seminal fluid by von Euler (1934). He thought they originated from the prostate and so gave them their name, though it is now known that the main source of prostaglandins in the seminal fluid is the seminal vesicles. Although they are found at their highest concentration in the seminal fluid, they have been isolated from many tissues, and can produce widespread effects in the body. A very large amount of research has been carried out on these compounds over the last 20 years, and it is now clear that a number of them are pharmacologically active on the muscle of the urinary tract.

Actions of Prostaglandins on the Urinary Tract Muscle

Of the different types of prostaglandins that have been described, those designated as PGE_1, PGE_2, $PGF_{1\alpha}$ and $PGF_{2\alpha}$ appear to be the ones which are active in the urinary tract. All have been shown to produce contractions of the bladder detrusor muscle in vitro (Abrams and Feneley 1976; Andersson et al. 1977). In the case of the human bladder, $PGF_{2\alpha}$ appears to be the most potent and PGE_1 the least potent in this respect, although there is some suggestion that there may be species differences in the degree of response. Many workers have stressed that the response, which is relatively powerful, develops more slowly and persists very much longer than does the response to acetylcholine. The effect on the human urethra of $PGF_{2\alpha}$ is to produce a contraction which is not affected by phenoxybenzamine, atropine or tetrodotoxin, whereas PGE_1 and PGE_2 produce relaxation which is greater than that produced by isoproterenol and is not affected by propranolol (Andersson et al. 1977). Here again there is some evidence of species differences, and the importance of caution in extrapolating the results of animal experiments to the human is clear.

With regard to the ureter, it has been shown that in the dog $PGF_{2\alpha}$ has a stimulatory effect (Boyarsky and Labay 1969) whereas PGE_1 has an inhibitory action (Wooster 1971). A comparable result has been reported in the case of the human ureter (Abrams and Feneley 1976), where despite some inconsistency there was a tendency for the PGE series to inhibit, and the PGF series to stimulate the contractions.

Whether the prostaglandins act directly on the urinary tract smooth muscle, or whether they produce their actions via specific receptors, is not yet decided. The facts that contrasting effects on anatomically contiguous muscles are found, that the stimulating effect is not abolished by papaverine, and that specific competitive blockade can be produced by the compound N-0164 (Khanna et al. 1978) all suggest that in the rabbit preparation at least, the effects are mediated via specific prostaglandin receptors. That receptors for some of the prostaglandins do indeed exist has been shown by ligand binding studies.

As has already been noted in Chap. 1 when discussing the purinergic nerves, there is experimental evidence that ATP-induced contraction of the rabbit detrusor may partly be mediated by local prostaglandin synthesis, and it is suggested that prostaglandins as well as ATP may contribute to the non-adrenergic non-cholinergic component of bladder contraction (Andersson et al. 1980).

Production of Prostaglandins in the Urinary Tract

Not only do the prostaglandins produce an effect on the urinary tract musculature, but there is also evidence that they are themselves produced in the tissues, and it has been suggested that the prostaglandins are not stored but are synthesised locally as required. Bultitude et al. (1976) concluded from their experiments on both animal and human bladder strips that there is a spontaneous production of PGE_2. Khalaf et al. (1979) found in dog experiments that there is a significant release of prostaglandins into the pelvic venous blood in response to both bladder distension and pelvic nerve stimulation, and in a later publication (Khalaf et al. 1980) they showed that prostaglandins are secreted into the lumen of the bladder, and that the low resting level rises after both micturition and pelvic nerve stimulation. Abrams et al. (1979) have shown that human detrusor strips produce both PGE and PGF, particularly the former. It has been suggested that the prostaglandins, perhaps particularly PGE_2, play a role in the maintenance of bladder tone during filling (Poggesi et al. 1980).

There is good evidence that the human prostate itself produces prostaglandins, and Cavanaugh et al. (1980) showed that both the production and the metabolism of $PGF_{2\alpha}$ by the human prostate are increased by androgens and by lactogen. In the case of benign enlargement of the prostate, Rolland et al. (1981) have produced evidence that PGE_2 is produced in or adjacent to the gland.

Therapeutic Applications

Prostaglandins

Because of their demonstrable actions on the urinary tract, a number of attempts to use the prostaglandins for therapeutic purposes have been reported, principally in cases in which difficult micturition and poor or absent bladder contractility are the problem. Logically, from what has been outlined above, PGE_2, which causes contraction of the detrusor without a similar contraction of, or possibly even with relaxation of, the posterior urethra, would be the prostaglandin of choice. $PGF_{2\alpha}$, although a more powerful detrusor stimulant, would have the disadvantage of simultaneously contracting the posterior urethra.

In clinical trials the prostaglandins have been administered locally by bladder instillations or in the form of an intra-urethral jelly. Several authors have reported encouraging results with the prostaglandins themselves (Bultitude et al. 1976; Andersson et al. 1978; Desmond et al. 1980). More recently, Vaidyanathan et al. (1981) have reported some success with the 15(S)-15 methyl analogue of $PGF_{2\alpha}$ in improving voiding in patients with neurogenic bladder dysfunction. This agent has a longer half-life and a greater potency than $PGF_{2\alpha}$ itself. These authors, as have others before them, remarked on the prolonged benefit (up to 2½ months) experienced by some of their patients. In contrast to these encouraging reports it must be noted that others (e.g. Delaere et al. 1981b) have failed to obtain any reliable evidence of a beneficial effect, and this mode of treatment must at present be regarded as still experimental.

Prostaglandin Antagonists and Inhibitors

A few substances have been described which have a blocking effect on the actions of prostaglandins on certain cells. These include the compound N-0164 mentioned above (Eakins et al. 1976) and one designated SC-19220 (Sanner 1969). At present these do not have any practical clinical importance.

In contrast to these blockers, drugs which inhibit the synthesis of prostaglandins are well known and are widely used in clinical practice, and some of them have been employed for the treatment of urinary tract disorders. It has been postulated that one of the factors involved in the unstable detrusor, whether idiopathic or neurogenic, could in some way be related to the local production and action of the prostaglandins. Accordingly, attempts to inhibit the production of prostaglandins with the synthetase inhibitors have been made in this condition. Good results with indomethacin were reported by Cardozo and Stanton (1980), whereas Delaere et al. (1981a), in a series of 55 patients with idiopathic detrusor instability, were not able to show any significant benefit with oral administration. Cardozo et al. (1980) used flurbiprofen, a propionic acid derivative related to ibuprofen (Brufen) which is reputed to be about 20 times more active than indomethacin, and obtained a significant improvement in the symptoms of frequency, urgency and urge incontinence, as well as in the objective cystometrogram findings, in a double-blind placebo cross-over study of 30 women.

Prostaglandin synthetase inhibitors have also been used therapeutically for a possible effect on the ureter, particularly in an attempt to relieve ureteric colic. Encouraging results were reported with indomethacin administered intravenously (Holmlund and Sjödin 1978), and more recently with a relatively new synthetase inhibitor, diclofenac sodium (Voltaren), administered intramuscularly (Lundstam et al. 1980). However, the possibility must be considered that the beneficial clinical effects may be due to mechanisms other than a direct effect on the ureteric muscle. It is known that synthesis of PGE_2 in the kidney is normally stimulated by a rise in pressure in the renal pelvis, and this results in an increased renal blood flow. In a recent paper Sjödin and Holmlund (1982) have reported experimental work which suggests that the prostaglandin synthetase inhibitors may act on this mechanism, inhibiting the production of the PGE_2, thus reducing the intrapelvic and intra-ureteric pressure in the case of an obstructed ureter, and hence reducing the pain.

Conclusions

One of the drawbacks with the prostaglandin synthetase inhibitors tried so far is that they have pronounced side-effects which seriously limit their use. At present, it must be concluded that the prostaglandins and their allied drugs are not of practical therapeutic value in urology. However, it seems likely that, with the enormous amount of interest and research that is continuing in the subject of the prostaglandins, further developments could well lead to the useful application in the field of urology of the prostaglandins themselves, their synthesis inhibitors, or their antagonists.

Histamine

Histamine has very widespread effects throughout the body, which are mediated via two types of receptors, designated as H_1 and H_2. The H_1 receptors are related to the contractile effect produced on smooth muscle, as is seen particularly in the smooth muscle of the bronchi and of the gastro-intestinal tract, whereas the H_2 receptors are those mediating the stimulatory action of histamine on the gastric secretions. Both types of receptors appear to be involved in the vasodilation produced by histamine.

In the case of the smooth muscle of the urinary tract, investigations have indicated that H_1 receptors are present, but apparently no H_2 receptors. In vitro experiments on both animal and human muscle preparations show a powerful contractile response of the detrusor to histamine, with a lesser response of the urethra.

As would be expected from the type of receptor present, these contractions are abolished by H_1 blockers such as methapyriline and mepyramine, but are unaffected by the H_2 blockers such as burimamide and metiamide (Todd and Mack 1969; Khanna et al. 1977; Creed and Tulloch 1982). In the case of the ureter varying results have been reported, possibly due to species differences, but the majority seem to indicate a stimulatory effect, producing an increase in the resting tension and in the frequency and amplitude of the contractions.

The fact that atropine partially blocks the effects of histamine on the urinary tract has led to the suggestion that acetylcholine and muscarinic receptors may be involved in the mechanism of its action (Fredericks 1975), but not all authors agree with this (Khanna et al. 1977).

Although the above responses to histamine can be demonstrated experimentally, it is questionable whether this substance plays any role in the normal physiology of the urinary tract. It is possible that allergic reactions can manifest themselves in the urinary tract, and if this is the case then histamine is presumably involved.

The various widely used antihistamine drugs such as diphenhydramine (Benadryl) and tripelennamine (Pyribenzamine)), although they can be shown experimentally to block the effects of histamine, do not appear to produce any direct effect on the urinary tract via this mechanism. However, many of them also possess an anticholinergic action, and this may result in difficulty in micturition in patients to whom they are administered for the treatment of allergic conditions.

5-Hydroxytryptamine (Serotonin)

The amine 5-hydroxytryptamine is closely related to histamine, and produces a powerful contraction in both the animal and human bladder (Matsumura et al. 1968). In the ureter a wide variety of effects have been reported including stimulation, inhibition, initial inhibition followed by stimulation, and no effect at all.

In the case of the detrusor the effect produced has been shown to be biphasic, consisting of an initial transient contraction due to stimulation of the autonomic ganglia, followed by a more prolonged contraction due to a direct effect on the smooth muscle itself. At the same time, an additional opposing action due to inhibition of the parasympathetic ganglia exists (Saum and de Groat 1973). At present there is no evidence that these effects are of clinical importance.

Calcium Antagonists

Mode of Action

In the Introduction, when outlining some of the physiological events associated with the contraction of smooth muscle cells, reference was made to the fact that the necessary increase in intracellular calcium ions could be provided both by mobilisation of calcium from the intracellular stores such as the sarcoplasmic reticulum and the mitochondria, and by an increase in the net influx of ions into the cell via the calcium channels in the cell membrane. In recent years a new group of drugs has come into use whose specific action is generally accepted to be the inhibition of calcium entry through these channels (Fig. 2.2), especially those termed by Bolton (1979) the 'potential-sensitive ion channels'. Ziegler (1981), however, has recently questioned whether the action is truly on the ion channels, and has suggested that the underlying mechanism may rather be on the plasmalemmal stores, specifically an effect making the calcium less available from these. In either case, these drugs can cause a limitation of the availability of calcium ions for the contractile process, thus resulting in an inhibitory action on muscle contraction which is to a large extent independent of the mode of stimulation of the cell. The best known of these drugs are verapamil (Isoptin), nifedipine (Adalat) and terodiline, and although their main clinical uses to date

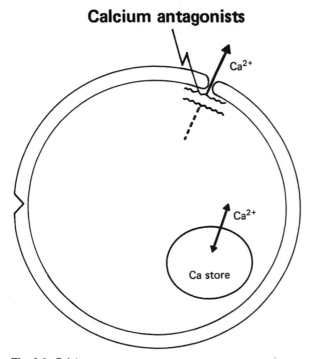

Fig. 2.2. Calcium antagonists inhibit entry of calcium ions (Ca^{2+}) via the cell membrane.

have been for their effects on the cardiovascular system, a number of observations have shown them to have an action on the smooth muscle of the urinary tract, which could prove to have some clinical value in urological practice.

Effects on the Urinary Tract

Experimental Effects

In the experimental animal, nifedipine has been shown to reduce the contraction of the electrically stimulated bladder by as much as 50%, whereas under the same experimental conditions verapamil had only a very weak effect in vitro and virtually none at all in vivo (Sjögren and Andersson 1979). In vitro studies of muscle taken from the human bladder, urethra and ureter showed that nifedipine produced an inhibitory effect on the responses to a variety of pharmacological agents including noradrenaline, prostaglandins, carbachol, potassium and barium chloride (Forman et al. 1978). Terodiline has been shown to have an inhibitory effect on the influx of calcium into smooth muscle (Østergaard et al. 1980), but in addition appears to have an antimuscarinic action which predominates at low concentration. In experimental studies on the rabbit bladder there seems to be a difference in its action from that of nifedipine, for whereas the latter abolishes the spontaneous activity of bladder strips, terodiline does not produce this effect, and may even augment the activity (Husted et al. 1980). In human bladder strips terodiline was found to inhibit carbachol-induced contractions. Whether this action is due to its muscarinic blocking effect or to its action as a calcium antagonist is not clear (Rud et al. 1980).

Experimental studies on the effect of verapamil on the rabbit bladder and proximal urethra have shown that it is capable of blocking the contractile effects of both acetylcholine and noradrenaline in a non-competitive fashion, and in higher concentrations it is also able to block contractions induced by ATP and calcium chloride. It was concluded that verapamil produces a non-selective blocking effect on both the neuroreceptor-mediated and the potential-mediated responses of smooth muscle (Khanna et al. 1982).

Clinical Effects

A few clinical studies have appeared, most of which report a beneficial effect of both nifedipine and terodiline in patients suffering from an unstable bladder detrusor. Nifedipine is said to reduce the frequency and amplitude of the uninhibited contractions shown on the cystometrogram, to increase bladder capacity, and to give symptomatic relief. There does not, however, appear to be any appreciable change in the resting tone of the bladder or of the urethra (Forman et al. 1978; Rud et al. 1979). The side-effects of nifedipine treatment, consisting mainly of tachycardia and a feeling of warmth in the face, are reported to be minimal. It must be noted, however, that not all authors agree with these findings, and Laval and Lutzeyer (1980) report that they were unable to find any significant effect of nifedipine on spontaneous bladder contractions in 30 patients with unstable detrusors.

Terodiline has been reported to produce both subjective symptomatic improvement and objective improvement in the cystometrograms in women suffering from urgency and urge incontinence due to an unstable detrusor (Rud et al. 1980; Ekman et al. 1980). In this case the question arises as to how much of the effect is due to the anticholinergic action, which as mentioned above is predominant at low concentrations. The fact that no other anticholinergic effects were experienced by these patients, unless the dose was doubled, led the authors to believe that the anticholinergic action alone did not account for the beneficial effects.

Phenothiazines

The phenothiazines are widely used in psychiatric practice, and a number of them such as chlorpromazine (Largactil), thioridazine (Melleril) and prochlorperazine (Stemetil) have been reported to have an effect on the function of the lower urinary tract. Experimental animal studies have indicated that these drugs can have a variety of modes of local action on smooth muscle, including a direct depressant effect, an antimuscarinic effect, and an alpha-adrenergic blocking action (Merrill and Markland 1970; Finkbeiner and Bissada 1979; Gilman et al. 1980). In addition, chlorpromazine has been shown to have an inhibitory action on the re-uptake of noradrenaline into the adrenergic nerve terminals (Tuck et al. 1972). Some of the effects of phenothiazines on micturition may also be related to their central cerebral actions.

Although these drugs are not used primarily for their actions on the lower urinary tract, their use for other purposes may produce untoward side-effects on micturition which the practitioner should be aware of. Two contrary types of reactions have been reported. In those cases where the predominant effect is on the bladder detrusor, difficulty in micturition and retention of urine can occur, presumably as a result of a combination of the antimuscarinic, direct muscle depressant, and possibly central actions (Merrill and Markland 1972), and such troublesome side-effects are by no means uncommon in patients with associated prostatic enlargement. In a few cases the effects are predominantly on the urethra, resulting in a diminished closure pressure and urinary incontinence. Such manifestations are most probably attributable to the alpha-adrenergic blocking properties, possibly together with a direct effect on the urethral muscle (van Putten et al. 1973).

Cardiac Glycosides

A beneficial action of digitalis on voiding difficulties in cardiac patients was noted by Sadoughi et al. (1973), and experimental studies have indicated that the digitalis glycosides can increase intravesical pressure and decrease bladder capacity in both humans (Sadoughi et al. 1975) and animals (Welch et al. 1975). The effect seems to be due to both a direct action on the muscle fibres, possibly as a result of inhibition of potassium–sodium-stimulated ATPase causing an increase in intracellular calcium ions, and a stimulatory action on the muscarinic cholinergic receptors (Bissada and Finkbeiner 1979).

The effects of ouabain, a related cardiac glycoside with a similar action to digitalis, have been studied on the ureter. Some results have indicated a biphasic action, with initial stimulation and subsequent decrease in excitability of the ureteric muscle reactions (Weiss et al. 1970), but others have found only an inhibitory effect, without any preliminary stimulation (Washizu 1968), the differences possibly being species related. No clinical effects on ureteric function in patients treated with the cardiac glycosides have been reported.

Narcotics

The question as to the pharmacological effects of the narcotic drugs such as morphine, papaveretum and pethidine is of interest and importance, because of their frequent use for painful conditions such as ureteric colic and bladder spasm. Many studies of the effects of these drugs on the ureter, both in humans and animals, have been carried out and have produced conflicting results. In the case of morphine and papaveretum the effects reported have varied from a stimulating action on both the tone and the peristaltic contractions (Macht 1916), through no effect at all (Weinberg and Maletta 1961; Struthers 1973), to a complete inhibition of the contractions (Ross and Griffiths 1970). Similarly, in the case of pethidine Struthers (1973) has reported a pronounced stimulating effect on the contractions, whereas Ross et al. (1972a) found either an inhibitory action or no effect at all.

In the case of the lower urinary tract similar contradictory findings have been reported, including a stimulatory effect or no effect on the detrusor with morphine (Edmunds and Roth 1920; Todd and Mack 1969), a reduction in intravesical pressure with papaveretum (Doyle and Briscoe 1976), and an inhibitory effect on the bladder and a rise in urethral pressure with pethidine (Doyle and Briscoe 1976). A number of reports of morphine apparently causing retention of urine have appeared in the literature.

Some of the discrepancies in the results obtained in the various investigations may be due to species differences, and some to inaccurate or fallacious methods of investigation. In the case of the ureter they may be related to variability in other parameters, such as the urine flow in the intact ureter, the presence or absence of continuity with a pace-maker, age, hormonal status, and so on. At present it does not seem to be possible to draw final conclusions from the results reported.

Anaesthetics

General and Epidural Anaesthetics

A number of the anaesthetic agents in common use have been shown to have a pharmacological effect upon the lower urinary tract. Doyle and Briscoe (1976) reported that both thiopentone and methohexitone (Brevital sodium) cause a particularly marked diminution of the urethral closure pressure. Epidural anaesthesia with bupivacaine up to the level of T6 also causes a reduction of the maximal urethral closure pressure in patients with benign prostatic enlargement, by an average of 44% (Appell et al. 1980). In this case, the anaesthesia presumably acts via the sympathetic nervous outflow rather than directly on the urethral muscle.

General anaesthetics have a depressant effect also on the bladder. Hill (1976) noted that both thiopentone and halothane reduced the response of strips of human detrusor to electrical stimulation, and concluded that this was due to a direct action on the muscle itself. Doyle and Briscoe (1976) found that halothane significantly reduced intravesical pressure during bladder filling, and often abolished abnormal detrusor contractions. A similar observation was made by Grossman et al. (1977), who found that uninhibited detrusor contractions in children were abolished by halothane anaesthesia. Nitrous oxide anaesthesia, on the other hand, did not abolish the contractions, although it sometimes slightly delayed their onset or diminished their intensity.

Observations such as the above may be of practical significance and importance. Not infrequently urodynamic and pharmacological studies, both in animals and in the human (particularly children), are carried out under anaesthesia, and it is clear that the investigator must be aware of any possible effects of the anaesthetic agents used, and must take these into account when assessing the results obtained.

Local Anaesthetics

Those local anaesthetics which possess a surface action are frequently used on the urethral and bladder mucosa as adjuncts to investigations and treatment of the lower urinary tract. The multitude of names employed for the same pharmacological agents leads to some confusion, but in practice there are two compounds which are in general use, namely lignocaine (Lidocaine, Xylocaine, Esracaine) and amethocaine (Tetracaine, Pantocain, Pontocaine, Decicain). The former is most commonly used in the form of a 2% urethral jelly to produce anaesthesia for procedures such as catheterisation, bouginage or endoscopy. The latter has a more powerful and prolonged action although it takes longer to reach its maximum effect, and hence is used in a lower concentration, such as 0.1%. It has been recommended as a mucosal anaesthetic for the bladder in cases of neurogenic dysfunction of the upper motor neuron type, in order to increase the capacity and reduce the uninhibited contractions, and has proved of prophylactic value in cases of autonomic dysreflexia. Higson et al. (1979) have reported that following intravesical instillation of 1% lignocaine there was a significant increase in bladder capacity, reduction in maximum detrusor pressure and reduction in bladder sensation in a group of patients suffering from detrusor instability. They used it together with an equal volume of 8.4% sodium bicarbonate solution, and stressed the importance of an alkaline environment. This increases the dissociation of the salt and the proportion of lipid-soluble free base which can diffuse more readily through the tissues.

In the case of the ureter, the local anaesthetics have generally been found to have an inhibitory effect on peristalsis, sometimes with an initial transitory stimulant action. Ross et al. (1972b) reported that the intraluminal injection of

2% lignocaine reduced peristaltic activity in 5 out of 15 ureters in their patients, and had no effect in the other 10. Andersson and Ulmsten (1975) found that local instillation of 4% lignocaine in their patients caused an initial brief stimulation followed by reduced activity. Tsuchida (1970) made electroureterogram studies of the dog ureter, and found that there was a prompt inhibitory effect of 4% lignocaine applied to the mucosa in vivo, whereas this was negligible when applied to the adventitia. In the case of the ureter studied in vitro, there was no difference between the two modes of application.

In contrast to these observations it must be recalled that Struthers (1976), in his in vivo studies in dogs, found that both systemic and intraluminal administration of lignocaine, procaine and mepivacaine caused only hyperperistalsis, and never inhibition. It is difficult to explain these discrepancies satisfactorily. It has been suggested that they may be due to variations in the effective concentrations of the drugs or the length of exposure to them, but there does not appear to be real evidence to support this. At present, there does not seem to be any practical clinical importance to the experimental findings with regard to the ureter.

References

Abrams PH, Feneley RCL (1976) The actions of prostaglandins on the smooth muscle of the human urinary tract in vitro. Br J Urol 47:909–915

Abrams PH, Sykes JAC, Rose AJ, Rogers AF (1979) The synthesis and release of prostaglandins by human urinary bladder muscle in vitro. Invest Urol 16:346–348

Andersson K-E, Ulmsten U (1975) Effects of spinal anaesthesia, lidocaine, and morphine, on the motility of the human ureter in vivo. Scand J Urol Nephrol 9:236–242

Andersson K-E, Ek A, Persson CGA (1977) Effects of prostaglandins on the isolated human bladder and urethra. Acta Physiol Scand 100:165–171

Andersson K-E, Henriksson L, Ulmsten U (1978) Effects of prostaglandin E$_2$ applied locally on intravesical and intraurethral pressures in women. Eur Urol 4:366–369

Andersson K-E, Husted S, Sjögren C (1980) Contribution of prostaglandins to the adenosine triphosphate-induced contraction of rabbit urinary bladder. Br J Pharmacol 70:443–452

Appell RA, England HR, Russell AR, McGuire EJ (1980) The effects of epidural anaesthesia on the urethral closure pressure profile in patients with prostatic enlargement. J Urol 124:410–411

Awad SA, Bryniak S, Downie JW, Bruce AW (1977) The treatment of the uninhibited bladder with dicyclomine. J Urol 117:161–163

Benson GS, Sarshik SA, Raezer DM, Wein AJ (1977) Bladder muscle contractility: comparative effects and mechanisms of action of atropine, propantheline, flavoxate and imipramine. Urology 9:31–35

Bissada NK, Finkbeiner AE (1979) In vitro action of digitalis on guinea pig detrusor and urethra. Invest Urol 17:1–2

Bolton TB (1979) Mechanisms of action of transmitters and other substances on smooth muscle. Physiol Rev 59:606–718

Boyarsky S, Labay P (1969) Ureteral motility. Annu Rev Med 20:383–394

Bradley DV, Cazort RJ (1970) Relief of bladder spasm by flavoxate. A comparative study. J Clin Pharmacol 10:65–68

Bultitude MI, Hills NH, Shuttleworth KED (1976) Clinical and experimental studies on the action of prostaglandins and their synthesis inhibitors on detrusor muscle in vitro and in vivo. Br J Urol 48:631–637

Cardozo LD, Stanton SL (1980) A comparison between bromocriptine and indomethacin in the treatment of detrusor instability. J Urol 123:399–401

Cardozo LD, Stanton SL, Robinson H, Hole D (1980) Evaluation of flurbiprofen in detrusor instability. Br Med J 280:281–282

Cavanaugh AH, Farnsworth WE, Griezerstein HB, Wojtowicz C (1980) The influence of testosterone and lactogen on synthesis and metabolism of prostaglandin $F_{2\alpha}$ by the human prostate. Life Sci 26:29–34

Creed KE, Tulloch AGS (1982) The action of imipramine on the lower urinary tract of the dog. Br J Urol 54:5–10

Delaere KPJ, Debruyne FMJ, Moonen WA (1981a) The use of indomethacin in the treatment of idiopathic bladder instability. Urol Int 36:124–127

Delaere KPJ, Thomas CMG, Moonen WA, Debruyne FMJ (1981b) The value of intravesical prostaglandin E_2 and $F_{2\alpha}$ in women with abnormalities of bladder emptying. Br J Urol 53:306–309

Desmond AD, Bultitude MI, Hills NH, Shuttleworth KED (1980) Clinical experience with intravesical prostaglandin E_2: Λ prospective study of 36 patients. Br J Urol 52:357–366

Diokno AC, Lapides J (1972) Oxybutynin: a new drug with analgesic and anticholinergic properties. J Urol 108:307–309

Doyle PT, Briscoe CE (1976) The effects of drugs and anaesthetic agents on the urinary bladder and sphincters. Br J Urol 48:329–335

Eakins KE, Rajadhyaksha V, Schroer R (1976) Prostaglandin antagonism by sodium p-benzyl-4-(1-oxo-2(4-chlorobenzyl)-3-phenylpropyl)phenylphosphonate (N-0164). Br J Pharmacol 58:333–339

Edmunds CW, Roth GB (1920) The point of attack of certain drugs acting on the periphery. I. Action on the bladder. J Pharmacol Exp Ther 15:189–199

Ekman G, Andersson K-E, Rud T, Ulmsten U (1980) A double-blind, cross-over study of the effects of terodiline in women with unstable bladder. Acta Pharmacol Toxicol (Kbh) 46 [Suppl] 1:39–43

Euler US von (1934) Zur Kenntnis der pharmakologischen Wirkungen von Nativsekreten und Extrakten männlicher accessorischer Geschlechtsdrüsen. Arch exp Pathol Pharmakol 175:78–84

Finkbeiner AE, Bissada NK (1979) In vitro study of phenothiazine effects on urinary bladder. Urology 14:206–208

Fischer CP, Diokno A, Lapides J (1978) The anticholinergic effect of dicyclomine hydrochloride in uninhibited neurogenic bladder dysfunction. J Urol 120:328–329

Forman A, Andersson K-E, Henriksson L, Rud T, Ulmsten U (1978) Effects of nifedipine on the smooth muscle of the human urinary tract in vitro and in vivo. Acta Pharmacol Toxicol 43:111–118

Fredericks CM (1975) Characterization of the rabbit detrusor response to histamine through pharmacologic antagonism. Pharmacology 13:5–11

Fredericks CM, Anderson GF, Kreulen DL (1975) A study of the anticholinergic and antispasmodic activity of oxybutynin (Ditropan) on rabbit detrusor. Invest Urol 12:317–319

Fredericks CM, Green RL, Anderson GF (1978) Comparative in vitro effects of imipramine, oxybutynin, and flavoxate on rabbit detrusor. Urology 12:487–491

Gilman AG, Goodman LS, Gilman A (1980) The pharmacological basis of therapeutics, 6th edn. Macmillan, New York Toronto London, p 403

Grossman HB, Koff SA, Diokno AC (1977) Cystometry in children. J Urol 117:646–648

Higson RH, Smith JC, Hills W (1979) Intravesical lignocaine and detrusor instability. Br J Urol 51:500–503

Hill DW (1976) Quoted by Doyle PT, Briscoe CE (1976) The effects of drugs and anaesthetic agents on the urinary bladder and sphincters. Br J Urol 48:334

Holmlund DE, Sjödin J-G (1978) Treatment of ureteral colic with intravenous indomethacin. J Urol 120:676–677

Husted S, Andersson K-E, Sommer L, Østergaard JR (1980) Anticholinergic and calcium antagonistic effects of terodiline in rabbit urinary bladder. Acta Pharmacol Toxicol (Kbh) 46[Suppl] 1:20–30

Johns A, Tasker JJ, Johnson CE, Theman MA, Paton DM (1976) The mechanism of action of dicyclomine hydrochloride on rabbit detrusor muscle and vas deferens. Arch Int Pharmacodyn Ther 224:109–113

Khalaf IM, Lehoux J-G, Elshawarby LA, Elhilali MM (1979) Release of prostaglandins into the pelvic venous blood of dogs in response to vesical distension and pelvic nerve stimulation. Invest Urol 17:244–247

Khalaf IM, Rioux F, Quirion R, Elhilali MM (1980) Intravesical prostaglandin: release and effect of bladder instillation on some micturition parameters. Br J Urol 52:351–356

Khanna OP, DiGregorio GJ, Sample RG, McMichael RF (1977) Histamine receptors in urethrovesical smooth muscle. Urology 10:375–381

Khanna OP, Barbieri EJ, McMichael RF (1978) Effects of prostaglandins on vesicourethral smooth muscle of rabbit. Urology 12:674–681

Khanna OP, DiGregorio GJ, Barbieri EJ, McMichael RF, Ruch E (1979) In vitro study of antispasmodic effects of dicyclomine hydrochloride on vesicourethral smooth muscle of guinea pig and rabbit. Urology 13:457–462

Khanna OP, Barbieri EJ, Moss M, Son D, McMichael R (1982) The effects of verapamil (calcium blocker) on the vesicourethral smooth muscle of rabbit. In: American Urological Association 77th Annual Meeting, pp 154–155 (Abstract 308)

Kohler FP, Morales PA (1968) Cystometric evaluation of flavoxate hydrochloride in normal and neurogenic bladders. J Urol 100:729–730

Laval K-U, Lutzeyer W (1980) Spontaneous phasic activity of the detrusor: a cause of uninhibited contractions in unstable bladders. Urol Int 35:182–187

Lundstam S, Wåhlander L, Kral JG (1980) Treatment of ureteral colic by prostaglandin synthetase inhibition with diclofenac sodium. Curr Ther Res 28:355–358

Macht DI (1916) On the pharmacology of the ureter. III. Action of the opium alkaloids. J Pharmacol Exp Ther 9:197–216

Matsumura S, Taira N, Hashimoto K (1968) The pharmacological behaviour of the urinary bladder and its vasculature of the dog. Tohoku J Exp Med 96:247–258

Merrill DC, Markland C (1970) A laboratory investigation of the effect of phenothiazines on urinary bladder function. Invest Urol 7:532–542

Merrill DC, Markland C (1972) Vesical dysfunction induced by the major tranquilizers. J Urol 107:769–771

Moisey CU, Stephenson TP, Brendler CB (1980) The urodynamic and subjective results of treatment of detrusor instability with oxybutynin chloride. Br J Urol 52:472–475

Østergaard JR, Østergaard K, Andersson K-E, Sommer L (1980) Calcium antagonistic effects of terodiline in rabbit aorta and human uterus. Acta Pharmacol Toxicol (Kbh) 46[Suppl] 1:12–19

Paulson DF (1978) Oxybutynin chloride in control of post-transurethral vesical pain and spasm. Urology 11:237–238

Paulson DF (1979) Oxybutynin chloride in the management of idiopathic detrusor instability. South Med J 72:374–375

Poggesi L, Nicita G, Castellani S, Selli C, Galanti G, Turini D, Masotti G (1980) The role of prostaglandins in the maintenance of the tone of the rabbit urinary bladder. Invest Urol 17:454–458

Putten T van, Malkin MD, Weiss MS (1973) Phenothiazine-induced stress incontinence. J Urol 109:625–626

Raz S, Zeigler M, Caine M (1972) Isometric studies on canine urethral musculature. Invest Urol 9:443–446

Rolland PH, Martin PM, Serment G, Roulier R, Rolland AM (1981) Human benign prostatic hypertrophy: role of prostaglandin E_2 and its relationships to bromocriptine therapy. Eur Urol 7:41–45

Ross JA, Griffiths JMT (1970) Morphine a spasmolytic? Br Med J III:107

Ross JA, Edmond P, Kirkland IS (1972a) Behaviour of the human ureter in health and disease. Churchill Livingstone, Edinburgh London, p 120

Ross JA, Edmond P, Kirkland IS (1972b) Ibid, p 125

Rud T, Andersson K-E, Ulmsten U (1979) Effects of nifedipine in women with unstable bladders. Urol Int 34:421–429

Rud T, Andersson K-E, Boye N, Ulmsten U (1980) Terodiline inhibition of human bladder contraction. Effects in vitro and in women with unstable bladder. Acta Pharmacol Toxicol (Kbh) 46[Suppl] 1:31–38

Sadoughi N, Tandoc V, Ablin RJ, Bush IM (1973) Effects of digitalis on urinary bladder. Urology 2:582–583

Sadoughi N, Razvi M, Ablin RJ, Bush IM (1975) The effects of digitalis on the bladder in man. J Urol 113:178–179

Sanner JH (1969) Antagonism of Prostaglandin E_2 by 1-acetyl-2(8-chloro-10,11-dihydrodibenz(b,f)(1,4)oxazepine-10-carbonyl)hydrazine (SC-19220). Arch Int Pharmacodyn Ther 180:46–56

Saum WR, de Groat WC (1973) The actions of 5-hydroxytryptamine on the urinary bladder and on vesical autonomic ganglia in the cat. J Pharmacol Exp Ther 185:70–83

Setnikar I, Ravasi MT, Da Re P (1960) Pharmacological properties of piperidinoethyl-3-methyl-flavone-8-carboxylate hydrochloride, a smooth muscle relaxant. J Pharmacol Exp Ther 130:356–363

Sjödin JG, Holmlund DEW (1982) Effects of saline load, roentgen contrast medium and indomethacin on diuresis and pelvic pressure in the acute obstructed kidney. An experimental study. Br J Urol 54:446–450

Sjögren C, Andersson K-E (1979) Effects of cholinoreceptor blocking drugs, adrenoceptor stimulants and calcium antagonists on the transmurally stimulated guinea pig urinary bladder in vitro and in vivo. Acta Pharmacol Toxicol 44:228–234

Stanton SL (1973) A comparison of emepronium bromide and flavoxate hydrochloride in the treatment of urinary incontinence. J Urol 110:529–532

Struthers NW (1973) An experimental model for evaluating drug effects on the ureter. Br J Urol 45:23–27

Struthers NW (1976) Modifications of ureteric peristalsis by local anaesthetic. An experimental study in dogs. Urol Res 4:151–155

Thompson IM, Lauvetz R (1976) Oxybutynin in bladder spasm, neurogenic bladder and enuresis. Urology 8:452–454

Todd JK, Mack AJ (1969) A study of human bladder detrusor muscle. Br J Urol 41:448–454

Tsuchida S (1970) Some factors controlling ureteral peristalsis. Tohoku J Exp Med 101:55–66

Tuck JR, Hamberger B, Sjöqvist F (1972) Uptake of ^{3}H-noradrenaline by adrenergic nerves of rat iris incubated in plasma from patients treated with various psychotropic drugs. Eur J Clin Pharmacol 4:212–216

Vaidyanathan S, Rao MS, Mapa MK, Bapna BC, Chary KSN, Swamy RP (1981) Study of intravesical instillation of 15(S)-15 methyl prostaglandin $F_{2\alpha}$ in patients with neurogenic bladder dysfunction. J Urol 126:81–85

Washizu Y (1968) Ouabain on excitation–contraction in guinea-pig ureter. Fed Proc 27:662

Weinberg SR, Maletta TJ (1961) Measurement of peristalsis of the ureter and its relation to drugs. JAMA 175:15–18

Weiss RM, Bassett AL, Hoffman BF (1970) Effect of ouabain on contractility of the isolated ureter. Invest Urol 8:161–169

Welch LT, Bissada NK, Redman JF (1975) Vesicotropic action of digitalis. Urology 5:361–364

Wooster MJ (1971) Effects of prostaglandin E_1 on dog ureter in vitro. J Physiol (Lond) 213:51P

Ziegler A (1981) On the mode of action of Ca-antagonists. Acta Pharmacol Toxicol (Kbh) 49[Suppl] 1:57

Chapter 3

Pharmacology of the Urinary Tract Striated Muscle

Marco Caine

Introduction

The previous two chapters have dealt mainly with the pharmacology of the smooth muscle which constitutes by far the greater part of the musculature in the urinary tract. However, it must be remembered that there is also a certain amount of striated muscle that is related to the outflow tract from the bladder. Pharmacological manipulation of this striated muscle is perhaps of less practical importance at the present time than that of the smooth muscle, partly because of the lack of any specificity of action of the drugs towards it. Nonetheless a number of pharmacological agents do have an action on it which can be of clinical value or of experimental importance. Before dealing with these, it is important to review briefly some of the present-day views on the relevant anatomy and physiology of this musculature.

Anatomy

In the past, the anatomy of the bladder outflow tract striated muscle was thought of in terms of the classically described external urethral sphincter situated in the pelvic floor, supplemented to some extent in its action by the levatores ani muscles, and receiving a somatic nerve supply via the pudendal nerve. Nevertheless, it has been realised for many years that striated muscle fibres can be found also in the wall of the urethra itself, from the level of the pelvic floor upwards.

With the recent developing interest in the pharmacology and neuroanatomy of the lower urinary tract, increasing evidence has accrued that the nerve supply to the striated muscle is not somatic alone, but that there are also autonomic sympathetic, and possibly parasympathetic, components (Donker et al. 1972; Elbadawi and Schenk 1974; Nanninga et al. 1977). Moreover, it has been noted on a number of occasions that although the striated muscle does to some extent respond as expected to neuromuscular blocking agents such as succinylcholine, this response, as also the response to pudendal nerve block, is incomplete (Petersén et al. 1961; Koyanagi 1980).

Gosling and his colleagues (Gosling and Dixon 1979; Gosling et al. 1981) have clarified the matter considerably in their recent publications. As the result of studies on human adult and fetal material, they have described two distinct striated muscle components. One, which they regard as the external urethral sphincter proper (the 'rhabdosphincter'), is situated in the wall of the urethra itself. In the female it forms a circular collar of striated fibres in the middle third of the urethra, closely applied to a thin layer of longitudinal smooth muscle fibres; in the male it is also intramural, in the region of the membranous urethra. This rhabdosphincter, according to their fetal dissections, receives its nerve supply from the pelvic plexus, and not from the pudendal nerve. Completely separated from this intramural sphincter by a continuous septum of connective tissue is what the authors refer to as the peri-urethral pelvic floor striated musculature, and this is supplied by the pudendal nerves. According to their light and electron microscopic studies, two different types of striated muscle are found in these tissues. One type, known as the 'slow twitch' or 'Type I', consists of specialised muscle fibres devoid of muscle spindles, which are capable of maintaining tone for prolonged periods without fatigue. The other fibres, known as 'fast twitch' or 'Type II' fibres, have a much larger diameter and different staining characteristics, and muscle spindles are present. These respond to stimulation with a rapid contraction. The intramural rhabdo-sphincter consists entirely of the Type I fibres, whereas the peri-urethral striated muscle contains both types of fibres, with a preponderance of Type I. According to these findings, therefore, one can envisage the intramural striated muscle as functioning as a sphincter, with maintained tone, an autonomic nerve supply, and probably a relative insensitivity to neuromuscular blocking agents. The peri-urethral striated musculature, whilst containing similar fibres, contains also Type II fibres which give it the property of rapid, forceful voluntary contraction controlled by the pudendal nerve.

Physiology

Unlike the condition obtaining in smooth muscle, the striated muscle cells are apparently supplied by only one motor nerve fibre each. The termination of the axon, after losing its myelin sheath, divides into a number of expansions known as terminal buttons, which are in intimate contact with a specialised thickened region of the muscle cell membrane referred to as the motor end-plate, but are separated from it by a synaptic cleft. The combined structure is known as a neuromuscular junction. Clear vesicles containing acetylcholine are present in the terminal buttons, comparable to those already described in the case of the cholinergic autonomic nerves, and, on the arrival of a nerve impulse, the acetylcholine is liberated from the vesicles into the synaptic cleft and unites with appropriate receptors on the motor end-plate. These receptors are classified as nicotinic in type, but in view of the difference in response of these receptors and the nicotinic receptors in the autonomic ganglia to the neuromuscular blockers and the ganglion blockers, it would appear that they are not identical. Stimulation of these receptors apparently alters the permeability of the membrane to sodium and potassium ions, as a result of which depolarisation occurs and an action potential is developed in the striated muscle cell. As in the case of the autonomic system, the liberated acetylcholine is probably rapidly deactivated by local anticholinesterase.

Drugs Acting on the Striated Muscle

Autonomic Drugs

Insofar as the rhabdosphincter has an autonomic nerve supply, one can anticipate a reaction to the autonomic drugs. The responses that have been reported appear to be limited to the alpha-adrenergic agonists and blockers, producing the expected corresponding increase and decrease in tone and closure pressure. No beta-adrenergic response has been obtained nor, despite the apparent identification of cholinergic fibres in histochemical studies (Elbadawi and Schenk 1974), has a cholinergic response been found (Koyanagi 1980) (see Fig. 1.7). However, because of the complexity of the tissues, it would seem extremely doubtful whether one could distinguish between the pharmacological responses of the smooth muscle and of the striated muscle, both types of muscle being found in very close apposition to each other in this region of the urethra.

Striated Muscle Relaxants

Paralysis or a low tone of the peri-urethral striated musculature will have little practical consequence as regards the normal control of micturition. It will affect only the 'active' component of continence, that is to say the active voluntary contraction of the muscle used to arrest the urinary stream; the 'passive' component, namely that responsible for the maintenance of continence at rest, will be unaffected (Caine and Edwards 1958). An excessively high tone or spasm of the muscle, on the other hand, or a failure of the normal reciprocal relaxation or 'external sphincter dyssynergia', as met with in supranuclear neurological lesions, can cause considerable interference with the urinary outflow. Although this condition is usually dealt with surgically, by transurethral external sphincterotomy or (less frequently today than in the past) by pudendal neurectomy, such modes of treatment have certain disadvantages such as the danger of impotence, incontinence, and occasionally troublesome operative haemorrhage. A satisfactory pharmacological alternative would therefore have advantages, and attempts to improve the condition by the use of drugs have been made, using principally the two striated muscle relaxants dantrolene sodium (Dantrium) and baclofen (Lioresal), and to a lesser extent the benzodiazepines (Young and Delwaide 1981).

Dantrolene

Dantrolene and baclofen, although both used specifically to relieve striated muscle spasm, have entirely different modes of action. Dantrolene acts on the muscle cell itself, beyond the neuromuscular junction, and is said to have more effect on the fast twitch type of muscle fibre than on the slow twitch type. It appears to suppress, but not completely inhibit, the intracellular release of calcium from the sarcoplasmic reticulum into the cytosol, as referred to in the Introduction. It does not seem to have any effect on the flux of calcium ions at the plasma membrane (Ellis and Carpenter 1974; Van Winkle 1976; Desmedt and Hainaut 1979) (Fig. 3.1).

A relaxant effect of dantrolene on the spastic striated muscle of the pelvic floor in cases of spinal cord injury has been demonstrated by a number of workers (Pedersen et al. 1978), and a measured reduction in the amount of residual urine and a diminution of electromyographic activity of the striated sphincter in 6 patients suffering from external sphincter hypertonicity of neuro-pathic origin was reported by Murdock et al. (1976). However, it seems to be only moderately effective, high doses are needed, and there may well be a risk of hepatic toxicity if such doses are used for prolonged periods (Hackler et al. 1980). There has been some suggestion that, experimentally, high doses of dantrolene may have a depressant effect also on smooth muscle (Graves et al. 1978), and Khalaf et al. (1979) reported a reduction in the resting intravesical

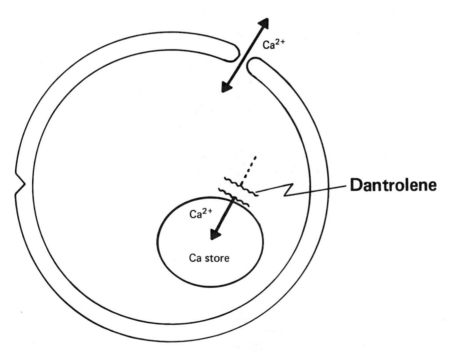

Fig. 3.1. Dantrolene is believed to act by suppressing the release of stored intracellular calcium ions (Ca^{2+}) into the cytosol. It does not affect their entry or exit at the plasma membrane.

pressure in the dog with high doses. This was in addition to a dose-dependent depression of the urethral pressure profile in the region of the striated sphincter, comparable to that produced by d-tubocurarine. However, other authors have not been able to confirm any effect on acetylcholine-induced contractions of the canine detrusor (Harris and Benson 1980). It does not have any appreciable effect on the ureter.

Baclofen

In contrast to dantrolene, baclofen does not have any action on the muscle cell itself, but acts on the reflex arc in the spinal cord. It is a derivative of gamma-aminobutyric acid (GABA), which is believed to be the natural mediator for presynaptic inhibition in the spinal cord, acting at the spinal ends of the upper motor neurons. Baclofen apparently acts in a similar manner, causing inhibition of the spinal cord reflexes, and is specifically of use in patients with spinal spasticity rather than those with spasticity of cerebral origin (Fig. 3.2). It may, in addition, reduce the release of excitatory transmitters, including the peptide called 'substance P', from nociceptive afferent nerve endings from the skin (Henry 1980). It has been shown to depress both the basic and the reflexly excited activity of the pelvic floor, including the external sphincter, in para-plegics and to a lesser extent in patients suffering from multiple sclerosis (Pedersen et al. 1974), as well as to reduce the urethral sphincter resistance and diminish residual urine in patients with spinal cord injuries (Leyson et al. 1980). In addition to its relaxant effect on striated muscle, Taylor and Bates (1979) found evidence of an effect on the primary unstable detrusor, resulting in a significant reduction in both diurnal and nocturnal frequency of micturition when compared with a placebo in a double-blind study. Similarly, Kiesswetter and Schober (1975) found it to be effective in reducing the detrusor hyper-reflexia in patients suffering from uninhibited neurogenic bladders due to spinal cord lesions, but not that due to cerebral lesions. In contrast to this, Hachen and Krucker (1977) found that intravenous baclofen produced a highly significant diminution of both sphincter pressure and residual urine in patients with upper motor neuron lesions of the bladder due to traumatic cord lesions, but were unable to demonstrate any effect on the detrusor.

In the cases of both baclofen and dantrolene, in the doses required to produce an effect on the striated muscle of the lower urinary tract, side-effects such as dizziness, drowsiness and increased generalised weakness are common and troublesome, and limit their usefulness.

Benzodiazepines

In addition to the above two drugs, the group of drugs known as the benzodia-zepines, although used mainly for their central tranquillising effects, are reputed to have a striated muscle relaxing action. The best known of this group are chlordiazepoxide (Librium), oxazepam (Serax), nitrazepam (Mogadon) and diazepam (Valium). The muscle relaxing action is believed to be due to an effect on the synapses of the spinal relfex arc, but these drugs, in contrast to baclofen, appear to act on the postsynaptic GABA receptors, increasing their sensitivity and thus causing a facilitation of potentiation of the inhibitory effect of the naturally occurring GABA (Fig. 3.2).

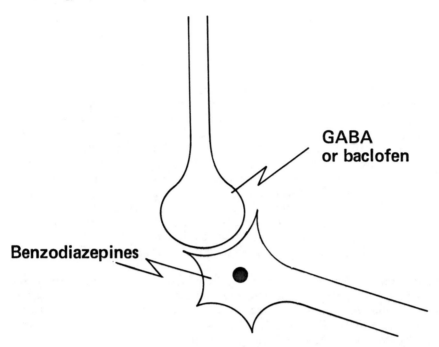

Fig. 3.2. It is believed that baclofen mimics naturally occurring GABA, inhibiting reflexes by acting at the spinal end of upper motor neurons. Benzodiazepines produce the same effect by increasing sensitivity of postsynaptic GABA receptors.

A small incidence of nocturnal enuresis developing in patients receiving diazepam or chlordiazepoxide was noted by Ditman and Gottlieb (1964). Diazepam has been reported to be of clinical value in improving bladder emptying in young women suffering from external sphincter spasm, when used together with the alpha-adrenergic antagonists phenoxybenzamine or methyldopa (Raz and Smith 1976), and Cook et al. (1977) reported that it produced an improvement in girls suffering from striated sphincter dyssynergia. In the cases in which these drugs appeared to have an effect on the striated muscle, however, it is not at all certain how much of this was truly an effect on the spinal reflexes and how much was simply due to their central cerebral effects. The fact is that in practice the sedative effects are often predominant, and may limit any potential usefulness for relieving striated urethral sphincter spasticity.

Neuromuscular blockers

In addition to those drugs acting on the striated muscle fibres themselves or on the spinal nervous pathways controlling them, there is a group of pharmacological agents which produce their effects by interfering with the activation of striated muscle at the neuromuscular junction. It is customary to divide these drugs, known as neuromuscular blockers, into two groups in accordance with what is known of their mode of action. One group, which includes *d*-tubocurarine (curare), gallamine (Flaxedil) and pancuronium (Pavulon), are known as 'competitive' or 'non-depolarising' blockers, and act by competing for and blocking the receptors on the motor end-plate. As mentioned earlier, these receptors are nicotinic in type, and this group of blockers also has a minor blocking effect on the nicotinic receptors in the autonomic ganglia. The other group, of which suxamethonium or succinylcholine (Scoline) is the best-known representative, are termed 'depolarising' blockers, and produce their effects by depolarising the cell membrane, resulting in lack of response to stimulation (Fig. 3.3). Suxamethonium produces an initial stimulation of the muscle cells, which is manifest as the fasciculation of the muscles fibres seen at the onset of its action, and its effect is terminated rapidly by breakdown by cholinesterase.

These drugs must be administered parenterally and are normally used only as adjuncts to general anaesthesia; hence their actions on the urinary tract may sometimes be difficult to differentiate from those of the anaesthetic agents themselves. Although they are not of therapeutic importance, their effects on the urinary tract musculature are of practical relevance with regard to both diagnostic and experimental procedures in which they may be used intentionally or incidentally, and therefore a brief review of their actions on the urinary tract will be given.

As their effects, especially those of the depolarising agents, are essentially on the striated muscle, they can be used to some extent to differentiate between the actions of this muscle and the smooth muscle in the bladder outflow tract, although reports on the effects produced are somewhat contradictory. Tanagho et al. (1969), for example, found that curare produced a drop of more than

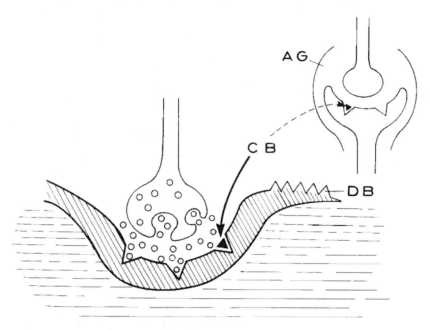

Fig. 3.3. Competitive neuromuscular blockers (CB) block nicotinic receptors on motor end-plates, and have a minor effect on receptors in autonomic ganglia (AG). Depolarising blockers (DB) have a direct action on the muscle cell membrane itself.

50% in the mid-urethral closure pressure in both humans and animals, as well as abolishing the effect of sacral nerve stimulation, and Awad and Downie (1976) found that gallamine reduced the peak urethral closure pressure in dogs, the effects in the male being more pronounced than those in the female. Doyle and Briscoe (1976), on the other hand, reported that they were unable to find any constant effect of neuromuscular blockers on the urethral pressure profiles of their patients. In considering these discrepancies the function of the somatically innervated striated muscle must be borne in mind, namely the development of an active voluntary contraction. It may be, therefore, that looking for variations in the resting urethral pressure profile (which reflects the tone of the muscle in a relaxed state), especially when the patient is under general anaesthesia, is not a reliable test for the blocking effect of these agents on the somatic neuromuscular transmission. Possibly such a blocking effect can only be assessed when the striated muscle is in a spastic state, as in the case of an upper motor neuron lesion, or when it is actively being stimulated to contract in response to nervous impulses.

There may be some difference in the urethral response to the two groups of agents because of the associated action of the competitive blockers on the ganglionic receptors, an action which is absent in the depolarising agents. This may explain the findings of Ghoneim et al. (1975) who noted that whereas after neuromuscular blockade with gallamine the normal reduction in urethral pressure in response to detrusor stretch was abolished, this was not the case after administration of succinylcholine. The sensitivity of all striated muscles to neuromuscular blockade is not identical, and there is some evidence that the urethral striated muscle may be relatively resistant. Thus Petersén et al. (1961) found the response of the urethral sphincter to intravenous succinylcholine to be appreciably less than that of the first interosseous muscle of the hand. It may well be that this difference can to some extent be accounted for by the autonomic component of the striated muscle nerve supply, which was not recognised at the time these findings were reported.

The possible effect of the neuromuscular blockers must be taken into account both in experimental work in vivo, and in relevant investigations in anaesthetised patients who have received such blockers. Their main clinical value in the urological field at present would appear to be in attempting to differentiate the somatic from the autonomic components in patients with abnormally high urethral closure pressures of neuropathic origin.

References

Awad SA, Downie JW (1976) Relative contributions of smooth and striated muscles to the canine urethral pressure profile. Br J Urol 48:347–354

Caine M, Edwards D (1958) The peripheral control of micturition: a cine-radiographic study. Br J Urol 30:34–42

Cook WA, Firlit CF, Stephens D, King LR (1977) Techniques and results of urodynamic evaluation of children. J Urol 117:346–349

Desmedt JE, Hainaut K (1979) Dantrolene and A23187 ionophore: specific action on calcium channels revealed by the aequorin method. Biochem Pharmacol 28:957–964

Ditman KS, Gottlieb L (1964) Transient enuresis from chlordiazepoxide and diazepam. Am J Psychol 120:910–911

Donker PJ, Ivanovici F, Noach EL (1972) Analyses of the urethral pressure profile by means of electromyography and the administration of drugs. Br J Urol 44:180–193

Doyle PT, Briscoe CE (1976) The effects of drugs and anaesthetic agents on the urinary bladder and sphincters. Br J Urol 48:329–335

Elbadawi A, Schenk EA (1974) A new theory of the innervation of bladder musculature. IV. Innervation of the vesicourethral junction and external urethral sphincter. J Urol 111:613–615

Ellis KO, Carpenter JF (1974) Mechanism of control of skeletal-muscle contraction by dantrolene sodium. Arch Phys Med Rehabil 55:362–369

Ghoneim MA, Fretin JA, Gagnon DJ, Susset JG (1975) The influence of vesical distension on urethral resistance to flow: the expulsion phase. Br J Urol 47:663–670

Gosling JA, Dixon JS (1979) Light and electron microscopic observations on the human external urethral sphincter. J Anat 129:216

Gosling JA, Dixon JS, Critchley HOD, Thompson S-A (1981) A comparative study of the human external sphincter and periurethral levator ani muscles. Br J Urol 53:35–41

Graves S, Dretchen KL, Kruger GO (1978) Dantrolene sodium: effects on smooth muscle. Eur J Pharmacol 47:29–35

Hachen HJ, Krucker V (1977) Clinical and laboratory assessment of the efficacy of baclofen (Lioresal) on urethral sphincter spasticity in patients with traumatic paraplegia. Eur Urol 3:237–240

Hackler RH, Broecker BH, Klein FA, Brady SM (1980) A clinical experience with dantrolene sodium for external urinary sphincter hypertonicity in spinal cord injured patients. J Urol 124:78–81

Harris JD, Benson GS (1980) Effect of dantrolene sodium on canine bladder contractility. Urology 16:229–231

Henry JL (1980) Pharmacologic studies on baclofen in the spinal cord of the cat. In: Feldman RG, Young RR, Koella WP (eds) Spasticity disordered motor control. Chicago, Year Book Publishers, pp 437–452

Kiesswetter H, Schober W (1975) Lioresal in the treatment of neurogenic bladder dysfunction. Urol Int 30:63–71

Khalaf IM, Foley G, Elhilali MM (1979) The effect of dantrium on the canine urethral pressure profile. Invest Urol 17:188–190

Koyanagi T (1980) Studies on the sphincteric system located distally in the urethra: the external urethral spincter revisited. J Urol 124:400–406

Leyson JFJ, Martin BF, Sporer A (1980) Baclofen in the treatment of detrusor-sphincter dyssynergia in spinal cord injury patients. J Urol 124:82–84

Murdock MM, Sax D, Krane RJ (1976) Use of dantrolene sodium in external sphincter spasm. Urology 8:133–137

Nanninga JB, Kaplan P, Lal S (1977) Effect of phentolamine on perineal muscle EMG activity in paraplegia. Br J Urol 49:537–539

Pedersen E, Arlien-Søborg P, Mai J (1974) The mode of action of the GABA derivative baclofen in human spasticity. Acta Neurol Scand 50:665–680

Pedersen E, Harving H, Klemar B (1978) Effect of dantrolene sodium on the spastic external urethral sphincter recorded by sphincterometry. J Urol 119:403–425

Petersén I, Kollberg S, Dhunér K-G (1961) The effect of the intravenous injection of succinylcholine on micturition: an electromyographic study. Br J Urol 33:392–396

Raz S, Smith RB (1976) External sphincter spasticity syndrome in female patients. J Urol 115:443–446

Tanagho EA, Meyers FH, Smith DR (1969) Urethral resistance: its components and implications. II. Striated muscle component. Invest Urol 7:195–205

Taylor MC, Bates CP (1979) A double-blind crossover trial of baclofen—a new treatment for the unstable bladder syndrome. Br J Urol 51:504–505

Van Winkle WB (1976) Calcium release from skeletal muscle sarcoplasmic reticulum: site of action of dantrolene sodium? Science 193:1130–1131

Young RR, Delwaide PJ (1981) Drug therapy—spasticity. New Engl J Med 304:28–33, 96–99

PART II

USE OF PHARMACOLOGICAL AGENTS IN URINARY TRACT DISORDERS

Chapter 4

Effects of Drugs on the Ureter and Renal Pelvis

Amos Shapiro and Saul Boyarsky

Rationale of Using Drugs in Ureteric Diseases

In this section we will, as far as possible, analyse the diseases of the ureter in terms of their pathophysiological elements, so as to enable a rational discussion of their drug therapy, and to distinguish therapy which is pharmacologically rational from that which is empirical. One must accept that sometimes empirical therapies are preferable to no therapy at all, but it must be borne in mind that the fact that the patient recovers or that his colic improves may or may not have been the result of the therapy. His recovery does not *prove* its efficacy, and certainly not the mechanism of its action, which is a scientific question. Conversely, many drugs which rationally should alleviate a patient's pain, may fail to do so for a variety of reasons, such as inadequate dosage, inadequate understanding of the relevant pharmacology, or the presence of secondary pathophysiological changes.

Despite the many drugs that have been used to treat ureteric diseases, ureteric pharmacology is still in its infancy and much research is still needed. Many uncontrolled and incompletely documented observations are to be found in the literature, and many of the basic observations made decades ago rest on techniques and methods considered today to be primitive. Advances in ureteric physiology since 1940 have shown certain recorded observations to have been defective and fallacious, particularly if the functional state of the ureter with regard to the quantity of urine flow had not been appropriately documented.

Standard authoritative texts of pharmacology, even the very best, have often uncritically repeated sweeping generalisations as to dosage, duration of activity, ureteric circulatory path, or influences on peristalsis, with no cognisance of the pharmacodynamics of the ureter itself. Some conclusions and generalisations have been derived from the pharmacology of the gut, arterioles, uterus or other organs, without any laboratory or clinical experience whatever. For instance, comments are made about the anticholinergic and antispasmodic effects of drugs on the ureter, but the role of cholinergic nerves in ureteric function remains obscure, and spasm in the ureter is a very vague concept. Such vagueness of the terminology reflects, in part, the uncritical and unsound conglomeration of the new and old literature.

A drug is useful in treating the ureter when it has a direct action on the pathological state, or a corrective and compensatory action on a relevant physiological state, so as to alleviate the effects of the disease being treated. However, there is no laboratory model which serves every purpose. For a drug to be clinically useful, it must reach the ureter in adequate concentration, must not disturb other tissues such as the heart, blood vessels, bowels or bronchi sufficiently to cause overpowering side-effects, and must influence the ureteric peristalsis or pathophysiological state at a safe dose and blood level. For many of the common drugs used to treat gastro-intestinal, cardiovascular, or uterine disorders, it is difficult to achieve a satisfactory dose level for the ureter without violating one of the above requirements.

The following factors influence ureteric peristalsis and may serve as pharmacological targets (Boyarsky and Labay 1972):

1) Hydrodynamic load, influenced by a) Obstruction, b) Diuresis, c) Bladder pressure and distension
2) Smooth muscle function, affected by such factors as a) Hyperkalaemia and hypokalaemia b) Hypocalcaemia c) Body temperature d) Neurohumoral control mechanisms acting on smooth muscle e) Certain smooth muscle drugs
3) Ureteric and 'renal' nerves a) Intrinsic b) Extrinsic c) Ganglia d) Sensory and motor apparatus e) Adrenergic and cholinergic (possibly histaminergic, serotonergic and other nerves?)
4) Hormonal a) Adrenal b) Posterior pituitary c) Oestrogenic and progestational steroids? d) Adrenal steroids? e) Prostaglandins?
5) Control mechanisms a) Hydrodynamic b) Neuromuscular, autonomic and central nervous system

From the standpoint of clinical medicine and surgery, the ureter has the following essential functional characteristics:

1) Patency or conduit function
2) Active peristalsis and propulsive function
3) Free gliding in its adventitial sheath, allowing non-restrictive peristalsis
4) Complete emptying, with no residual urine after contraction
5) Self-sterilisation, based in part on the above
6) Self-cleaning and emptying of particulate matter and encrustation

The ureter receives blood vessels, nerves and lymphatics, and glides in an adventitial sheath which has some of the characteristics of a serosal sheath. It is composed of three layers: epithelial, muscular and adventitial. The epithelial layer is an active cellular boundary between the tissue fluids and the urine which has been formed by the kidney, preventing reabsorption of urinary constituents. The muscle layer is intimately and complexly wound in an individual pattern for each level, and it is to this layer that the ureter owes its main function, that of propulsion by peristalsis of urine from the kidney to the bladder.

The anatomical relations of the ureter are important. However, it can also be the target of hormonal, biochemical, nervous and mechanical influences from distant organs. It is sensitive to hydrodynamic influences from within the urinary tract whether they be renal, ureteric or vesical.

Ureteric Physiology and Pathophysiology

The function of the ureter is to propel urine from the kidney to the bladder. Normally, the peristaltic impulse is generated in the most proximal portion of the collecting system, though whether in a single calix or several calices is not clear. A true pace-maker in the cardiac sense has never been identified but, physiologically, the generation of the impulse does have some of the characteristics of a pace-maker function. The impulse is conducted downwards along the renal pelvis, ureteric bulb and ureter ahead of the peristaltic muscular wave. These events are closely related to changes in cell membrane permeability and the internal and external ionic environments. Electrical changes have been described in association with fluxes of potassium, sodium and calcium. These electrophysiological and ionic phenomena suggest a potential target for drug therapy which has not been completely developed.

Experimentally, and occasionally clinically, a number of 'preparations' are available for observation and study. These include

1) The intact organism
2) Bladder explantation, produced experimentally or occurring naturally in the case of extrophy
3) The ureteric stump following nephrectomy
4) Diversion of urine through a pyelostomy
5) The effects of diuresis and antidiuresis
6) Bilateral adrenalectomy
7) Total renal and ureteric transplantation
8) Renal denervation
9) The ureter in other species

A wide range of techniques has been used in the laboratory to study the ureter, both in vivo and in vitro, in many different experimental animals, as well as in excised human tissues. Whereas previous generations have been limited to a large extent to such laboratory observations, modern radiographic, radioactive and surgical techniques currently permit more extensive observations to be made of human ureteric physiology. These include cinefluorography, needle aspirations and injections, computerised monitoring, three-dimensional biplane, and computerised tomography. These and similar sophisticated techniques have the effect of bringing the laboratory to the clinic.

Laboratory studies are directed almost entirely towards the peristalsis, and employ a variety of methods, such as

1) Morphological inference
2) Direct observation of the ureter at surgery
3) Plain film and intravenous urograms
4) Cinefluorography

5) Study of ureteric efflux at cystoscopy or after bladder explantation

6) Ureteric peristaltic pressure measurements

7) Ureteric perfusion through the pelvis or upper ureter

In addition, these methods can be supplemented by evidence from:

1) Tissue cultures

2) Biochemical assays, such as for catecholamines

3) Histological and histochemical studies, including neurohistochemistry

4) Total physiological monitoring

5) In vitro isotonic and isometric preparations for observing both the electro-physiological and the mechanical aspects of contractions

6) Inferences from dose–response curves to drugs

7) Biophysical computer models

8) Electromyography

Ureteric peristalsis above the point of lodgement of a stone may be suppressed, depending upon the duration and completeness of the obstruction. Such a decompensated or aperistaltic ureter results in an entirely different set of physiological conditions from the actively peristaltic ureter: its lumen communicates freely with the kidney and its physiological response may be blocked by the inertia and incompressibility of the trapped urine, so that no therapy may be effective until drainage has occurred. The force of urinary secretion pressure will be exerted directly against the calculus as long as renal function remains adequate. Such pressure may be stimulated and elevated by diuretics and renal haemodynamic changes. Once renal haemodynamics fail and hydronephrotic ischaemia develops, however, urinary secretion pressure begins to drop. This is a subacute process, requiring several days to a week to develop. The wall of the renal pelvis and ureter become stretched and flabby over a similar course of time.

The peristaltic changes developing during obstruction and diuresis should be recalled at this point. The antidiuretic and unobstructed ureter shows fairly regular small boluses and monophasic pressure waves, with complete closure and drop of intraluminal pressure between contractions. The midzone pattern of partial obstruction or early diuresis shows totally irregular waves with to-and-fro peristalsis, longer and more irregular boluses, and less emptying of the lumen. The obstructed ureter maintains a high intraluminal pressure with suppression of the discrete peristaltic waves, and with superimposed vascular pulsations transmitted from the renal artery.

Partial ligation and acute obstruction experiments show that the antidiuretic pattern may change to the completely obstructed type within several hours, depending upon the rate of urine flow and the length of ureter obstructed. However, in the partially or intermittently obstructed ureter, these changes will develop more gradually, because the ureter tends to buffer the kidney.

The highest pressures are achieved during acute distension of the ureter by a combination of diuresis and instrumentation due, apparently, to the stretch characteristics of the smooth muscle and the distension by incompressible fluid. In such situations, peak peristaltic pressures of 100 and 120 mmHg have been recorded in our laboratory, and confirmed by others. The maximum intraluminal pressure decays over a period of about 1 week.

Cinefluorographic visualisation during simulated 'colic' induced in the laboratory recapitulates the peristaltic changes of acute obstruction. A partially obstructed ureter, or a completely obstructed ureter in the first 30–60 minutes, shows bolus slowing, hesitation or reflection. Dilation and pools may form above the calculus, and the bolus may be reflected back upwards, so as to distend the pelvis and calices in a water hammer effect. To-and-fro waves, turbulence, luminal distension and eventually ineffective peristaltis, coiling and tortuosity and cessation of all movement follow as the obstruction increases.

Sites of Drug Actions

The sites of drug action affecting the pelvis and ureter can be classified anatomically. This classification may relate to the gross anatomy, including such divisions as the renal pelvis, various levels of the ureter, the uretero-vesical junction, etc., as well as the central nervous system, autonomic nervous chain and adrenal gland. It may relate to the finer anatomy, such as the ureteric muscle spirals, the blood vessels, lymphatics and nerves. Or it may relate to the level of the cells and their components, such as the cell membranes, intracellular systems, enzyme systems, specific systems and specific ions.

Any organelle, level of organisation, physiological parameter or pathological process may be the locus of action for a drug. Receptors and effector mechanisms may be shared with other tissues and organs. One must note that the method by which an observation was made influences the response and, hence, our 'facts' and theories.

Posology

The route of administration of a drug governs its rate of absorption and distribution. Immediately after administration, drug dissipation, transformation, destruction and excretion begin. The effect of the drug depends on its final concentration at the receptor site.

Responses occur after a threshold concentration is reached, and their direction may vary with the state of the receptor. There may be a reversal of the direction of drug effect, depending upon the time after administration at which it is observed, the method used, the ureteric parameter measured, and the ureter's functional state. Because words are inadequate to describe pharmacology and may produce paradoxes and contradictions, we rely upon the tools of science: mathematics, graphs, concepts, models, computers and statistics. Drug actions are thus best described in terms of a dose–response curve for each species, functional state, preparation and method.

Each drug which affects the ureter indicates a receptor and a site and mode of action. It also forms part of a pharmacological classification, the theory behind which further elucidates physiology and clinical medicine. A drug may also represent a family of compounds whose molecular biology points to a biological lock for its particular key. And finally, a drug may have an effect on other organs, the responses of which could aid in understanding its actions, even though clinically the result is undesirable side-effects.

In striving toward a ureteric pharmacology, the above philosophy of research is offered as a suggestion and guide to future workers, with the hope they may learn from our mistakes and false starts, when they utilise newer techniques and methods. They will need to understand progress made in the past and recognise the relevance of the older literature to the problems of their time.

The Use of Drugs in Ureteric Diseases

In this section the drugs acting on the ureter are described according to their action on ureteric disease, rather than their pharmacological or physiological classifications. Ureteric diseases may be classified on an aetiological basis in the following manner:

1) Obstructive
2) Calculous
3) Vascular: extrinsic and intrinsic
4) Metabolic
5) Degenerative
6) Nervous
7) Inflammatory, including tuberculous
8) Traumatic, including irradiation
9) Neoplastic
10) Congenital, genetic and enzymatic
11) Endocrine

They have not been systematically analysed in this manner. The common ureteric diseases such as colic due to stone, and subacute and chronic obstructions typified by tuberculosis, retroperitoneal fibrosis, strictures, endometriosis and transitional cell carcinoma are discussed. Conditions in which impaired peristalsis, rather than obstruction, is believed to be the main disturbance, such as pelvo-ureteric junction and vesico-ureteric junction obstructions, megaureter, pregnancy, and the effects of contraceptive pills are then dealt with. Drugs which may, as judged by reports in the research literature, be useful in the future but are still clinically unproven are also mentioned.

Ureteric Colic

The treatment of ureteric colic represents the commonest clinical use of drugs in ureteric disease. Since so many other ureteric conditions contain an obstructive element, this will also serve as a baseline for subsequent discussions.

The pathophysiological changes associated with ureteric colic include disordered peristalsis, obstruction to the secretion of urine, distension and dilation of the lumen and stretching of the wall, muscular hypotonia and paralysis, an inflammatory response in the wall of the ureter, pain, and reflex changes secondary to the pain, obstruction and mural involvement. It is usually a manifestation of the passage of a calculus and ureteric obstruction, but may also be caused by a blood clot, a sloughed papilla, other particulate matter, and more rarely by a sudden diuresis in the face of partial obstruction (so-called intermittent hydronephrosis). The mechanism of production of the pain and colic is considered to be due to a rapid rise in peristaltic or intraluminal pressure, with stretching of the ureteric wall innervated by thoracic 11, thoracic 12 and lumbar 1 segments (Davis et al. 1981). Increased intraluminal pressure first produces hyperperistalsis, then disordered peristalsis and, lastly, an aperistaltic state; urine production fails slowly, the urine composition changes and renal clearances diminish. Vascular and lymphatic readjustments also occur (Risholm 1954). The inflammatory changes in the ureteric mucosa are first those of oedema and exudation. Subsequently, the entire wall and peri-ureteric tissues become involved, with chronic lymphoedema, thickening, and then granulomatous, proliferative and fibrotic changes.

The therapy of ureteric colic is directed first to an accurate diagnosis, particularly in terms of ascertaining its cause, quantitating the degree of obstruction, and detecting any coexisting infection which would require immediate drainage and bacteriological therapy. Relief of pain and facilitation of the passage of the calculus come next. Recent work has suggested that aspirin and the steroidal and non-steroidal anti-inflammatory drugs have a salutary effect upon the oedema and mural inflammation, and will prevent or minimise subsequent proliferative and cicatricial changes which interfere with passage of the stone (Holmlund and Hassler 1965). The most useful drugs in relieving the pain of renal colic are as follows:

Meperidine (Dolestin; Demerol; Pethidine). Meperidine is a potent analgesic alkaloid which acts on the central and peripheral nervous systems to relieve pain. It has been reported by Struthers (1973) to increase the peristaltic rate after intravenous injection in the dog, in a manner similar to morphine. On the other hand, Kinn et al. (1982) showed that pethidine and norpethidine relax the smooth muscle of human hydronephrotic pelves. With the renewed interest in the action of the endorphins, a whole area of research in these drugs may open.

Pethidine is given intravenously up to 100 mg per treatment, in a slow injection until the pain is relieved. Usually 50–75 mg are sufficient, and treatment can be repeated several times a day.

Dipyrone (Optalgin). Dipyrone is a potent antipyretic, analgesic and anti-inflammatory drug widely used outside the USA in treating renal colic, especially in combined action with papaverine. The regime of 1–2 g of dipyrone, and 80 mg of papaverine intravenously every 3–5 hours has proved to be a very effective treatment in the experience of one of us (A.S.). This drug is seldom used in the USA for fear of agranulocytosis.

Papaverine. The alkaloid papaverine is a smooth muscle relaxant with a direct effect on the muscle. It increases the concentration of cyclic AMP and potentiates beta-adrenergic-mediated ureteric relaxation (Gruber 1928). Few pharmacological studies exist, and no controlled clinical studies have proved what remains to date a distinct clinical impression, namely a beneficial effect in relieving ureteric colic. Here is another fertile area for clinical and basic research.

Clinically, the factors considered to influence the spontaneous passage of ureteric calculi are:

1) The presence or absence of ureteric peristalsis
2) The size and shape of the calculus
3) The hydrostatic pressure generated by the obstruction
4) The time interval during which these factors are operating

To treat the disordered peristalsis of colic pharmacodynamically requires more perceptive methods and concepts than are used clinically today, so as firstly to describe the peristaltic abnormalities and, secondly, to select the appropriate drug to modulate the disordered peristalsis back to one producing an effective propulsion and expulsion of the stone. Preliminary studies in a dog model have shown how much more complex the disorder is than is envisaged by the usual clinical concept (Kim et al. 1970). Therapy in ureteric colic should not be based upon an oversimplified theory of pipe flow. The poor showing of pharmacological therapy for colic has been largely, though not entirely, a reflection of the poor understanding of the disorder, leading to a poor choice of therapeutic agents and selection of indications.

The concept of colic compiled from the experimental literature by Kim and his co-workers (1970) suggests that the following reactions to ureteric obstruction by a calculus occur:

1) Renal function responds to altered peristalsis, rising pelvic pressure and sustained obstruction by changes in haemodynamics, urine composition, clearances, nephron flows and tissue composition, which may differ for each type of molecular species and each particular renal function.
2) The upper ureter and renal pelvis function differently from normal during intermittent, partial or complete sustained obstruction.
3) The ureteric wall adjacent to an impacted calculus responds with inflammation, oedema, proliferative changes, fibrosis and external scarring.
4) The ureter below the obstruction, insofar as its urinary load is diminished and the conduction of impulses to it is altered, becomes relatively inactive, but does not lose its capacity for activity.
5) The contained urine may be altered by continued secretion during obstruction, inflammatory exudation into the lumen, and reabsorption from backflow and extravasation along the routes of urinary backflow (the fornices of the calices, and the renal and ureteric lymphatics leading into the perirenal and peri-ureteric spaces in the retroperitoneum).
6) The response of the autonomic nervous system, spinal cord and brain, and the psychological reaction of the individual to obstruction must be taken into account. These may result in reflex effects in other viscera and systems, such as the contralateral kidney and ureter; and physiological, psychological and behavioural responses to the pain.
7) It is possible that other responses will be discovered.

The response of the ureteric wall to a calculus has not received a great deal of attention. The literature supports the impression that anti-inflammatory therapy such as antibacterial or enzymatic medication can facilitate the passage of calculi. Inflammatory oedema of the ureteric wall due to manipulation or trauma is well known, and its progression to proliferative cicatricial and peri-ureteric changes is established. Extraluminal extravasation and reabsorption, retroperitoneal oedema and fibrosis and spontaneous extravasation of urine during colic have been described.

In confirmation of the earlier literature, Holmlund (1968) has reported a controlled series in which anti-inflammatory treatment of colic patients improved the rate and the speed of stone passage. Nevertheless, forcing fluids or inducing a diuresis in order to elevate intraluminal pressure, should renal function survive the acute insult, is accepted to be a legitimate mode of therapy and is an extremely popular one, although periodically questioned. Treatment of hyperperistalsis by the use of alpha-adrenergic blocking agents has been reported to be helpful in a series published by Kubacz and Catchpole (1972). Many patients with colic have presumably been obstructed long enough to have reached an aperistaltic state. Treatment with glucagon, which produces diuresis and aperistalsis in the dog model, has been disappointing in a short series of controlled studies, in spite of initial enthusiastic reports of success and the apparently good rationale.

A great potential exists for research in this area now that modern imaging techniques facilitate the visualisation of the ureter. One principle requires repetition: that the drug therapy of ureteric colic is adjunctive to cystoscopic and surgical therapy, and a properly managed patient is one who is closely monitored with all options immediately available.

Other drugs which are used for pain control of ureteric colic, but with limited experience, are:

Morphine. According to the older literature morphine increases the amplitude and frequency of peristalsis in vitro in high concentrations. Data are from various species, including the human (Gruber 1928; Marsala 1980). With the recent advent of epidural morphine administration for segmental anaesthesia, this drug has been used successfully in 5 cases of intractable colic due to stone obstruction, producing rapid expulsion and pain relief (Olshwang et al. 1984).

Butorphanol. Butorphanol is a synthetic product with analgesic properties. It is one of the iminoethanophenanthrene class of drugs, is five times more potent than morphine, is rapidly acting both intravenously and intramuscularly, has reported withdrawal symptoms, and a mild spasmogenic effect on smooth muscle. Its activity in ureteric colic was compared with that of meperidine by Elliott et al. (1979). Two milligrams of butorphanol had an effect equal to 80 mg of meperidine, and a butorphanol dose of 4 mg was superior for pain relief.

Lignocaine (Lidocaine; Xylocaine). Local use of Lidocaine and its cogeners can produce ureteric relaxation. The urothelium absorbs these materials. Locally applied to the ureter, they cause complete anaesthesia and reduced peristaltic rate (Borgstedt 1960). On the other hand, small amounts of Xylocaine can stimulate peristalsis and produce retrograde peristalsis when applied to the area of the vesico-ureteric junction (Shiratori and Kinoshita 1961). This class of drug may prove useful in the treatment of renal colic with pre-existing nephrostomies, or other access to the lumen of the kidney or ureter.

Subacute and Chronic Obstruction

Subacute and chronic obstructions are produced by post-inflammatory, post-surgical and post-infectious strictures, by tuberculosis, and by certain neoplasms. The pathophysiology includes constriction of the lumen, rigidity of the ureteric wall, fixation of the ureter by external traction adhesions, peristaltic pressure changes in the upper ureter, pelvis and calices and, eventually, changes in the gross morphology of the kidney, renal lymphatics, renal clearances and haemodynamics. From the standpoint of drug therapy, the volume of urinary secretion and the peristalsis of the muscle above the strictured ureter receive attention.

These obstructions tend to be slowly progressive. Diagnosis needs to specify (1) level, (2) duration, (3) degree of obstruction, (4) bilaterality, and (5) renal functional impairment. The most serious complication, that of infection, adds a potentially fulminant component to the disease and must receive first priority, requiring immediate cystoscopic or surgical drainage.

Tuberculosis

Tuberculosis can be complicated by strictures at various sites from the calices to the bladder. To prevent that complication, steroids are advocated in addition to triple drug treatment.

Prednisone (Meticorten). This adrenal cortical steroid is used to prevent the formation of ureteric stricture in tuberculosis. A 75% success rate has been reported if it is used before the stricture has worsened (Hallwachs and Baar 1972; Caine 1981). The recommended mode of treatment is an initial dosage of 30 mg a day for several months, with a gradual reduction of dosage subsequently.

Retroperitoneal Fibrosis

Retroperitoneal fibrosis is a condition which fascinates urologists since the externally trapped ureter does not show the completely obstructed lumen which its accompanying severe renal obstruction and failure would suggest. These ureters are often easily catheterised. They show the degree of obstruction and renal failure which can result from trapping long lengths of the ureter by external adventitial adhesive bands. The treatment is discussed in Chap. 8.

Endometriosis and Pregnancy

Endometriosis and pregnancy produce their effects mainly by mechanical compression of the ureter, although there is evidence in pregnancy and a remote suggestion in endometriosis, that the ureter may have been conditioned to show greater distensibility due to progestational changes.

Danazol. Danazol is a synthetic derivative of ethynyl testosterone, which suppresses ovarian function by decreasing gonadotrophins and luteinising hormone secretion. It suppresses endometrial development. Gardner and Whitaker (1981) treated two cases of endometriosis of the ureter successfully with this drug, using a dosage of 200 mg daily for one year.

Isolated case reports have suggested that ureteric dilatation has followed the use of the contraceptive pill, but they remain surmises, since most women taking birth control pills do not manifest such a hydroureter nor hydronephrosis. The bulk of the evidence clearly favours a mechanical cause for the hydronephrosis of pregnancy in humans.

All in all, a rational pharmacotherapy of the subacutely and chronically obstructed ureter has been hampered by lack of a clinical methodology for describing the pathophysiology of the ureter accurately.

Neoplastic Disease

Recurrent neoplastic disease of the ureter can cause severe obstruction, and a combination of cytotoxic drugs is recommended.

Cytotoxic Drugs. CISCA (*cis*-platinum, cyclophosphamide, doxorubicin), and FAM (5FU, doxorubicin, mitomycin C) have been reported in 7 patients with recurrent or metastatic transitional cell carcinoma of the renal pelvis to produce improvement in survival and remission time. Isolated reports on fewer cases with partial success of the use of cyclophosphamide and *cis*-platinum (Yagoda et al. 1978) and CISCA (Sternberg et al. 1977) were also encouraging. We are approaching an era of chemotherapy for the treatment of secondary ureteric tumour, as more effective agents evolve.

Impaired Peristalsis

This category of ureteric disease includes two elements, one demonstrable and the second postulated. The former is the dilatation of the proximal system above a lesion. The latter is the postulated lesion required to explain non-obstructive dilatation, as seen in megaureter, which is a poorly understood condition with dilatation, stasis, impaired peristalsis and atony. Pelvi-ureteric junction dysfunction, vesico-ureteric junction dysfunction and vesico-ureteric reflux may also belong in this category.

In this mixed category of diseases peristaltic contraction can be impaired, and smooth muscle stimulating drugs may prove to be helpful, particularly where surgery is contraindicated or unnecessary by virtue of the slow progression of the disease and lack of deterioration in renal function. Currently, however, management is either by surgery or by mere observation.

Clinically Available Drugs with a Known Effect on the Ureter

As our understanding of the complexity of ureteric peristalsis has improved, a range of drugs with a potential impact on ureteric peristalsis and its pathophysiology has emerged from the pharmacopoeia of the heart, uterus, bowel and blood vessel. It is only the lack of economic resources which restricts basic research in this field, for the literature is replete with suggestions of possible drug effects on the ureter. The dream of a 'digitalis' to improve the functioning of the ureter, as the cardiac glycosides did for the failing heart, is one such suggestion. The use of metoclopramide (Primperan) a procainamide derivative, is one such recent addition to the clinical armamentarium that was suggested by animal experiments. Although most of the drugs in this group do not at present have any practical clinical application, this may well change in the future. A brief account of them and their pharmacological effects upon the ureter is therefore desirable.

Sympathomimetic Agents

Noradrenaline. Noradrenaline is generally classified as an adrenergic agonist which serves as the major transmitter of the sympathetic system at the neuro-muscular junction. It has an excitatory effect on the ureter by activation of the alpha-adrenergic receptors, increasing the amplitude and frequency of contrac-tions in the human, rat, dog, pig and guinea-pig ureters in vitro (Malin et al. 1968, 1970; Weiss et al. 1978). This effect extends to the caliceal system and the renal pelvis. Experiments in vivo showed excitation of the quiescent ureter after administration of noradrenaline. The effect can be blocked by the approp-riate, specific blocking agent. On the other hand, blocking the beta receptors so as to leave the alpha receptors unopposed, markedly increases the effect of noradrenaline on the ureter (Weiss et al. 1978). Although noradrenaline has not been used to treat ureteric diseases, the theoretical importance of this drug is great in suggesting a whole line of second and third generation drugs for the ureter.

Ephedrine. Ephedrine is classified by pharmacologists as both an alpha- and a beta-adrenergic stimulator. It has a direct action on these receptors by displacing endogenous catecholamines from their granules in the adrenergic nerve endings, as do the amphetamines. It acts like adrenaline on the ureter. A high concentr-ation of ephedrine decreases ureteric peristalsis and tension (Vereecken 1973). It has had no application in the clinical treatment of ureteric diseases.

Phenylephrine (Neosynephrine). Phenylephrine is classically a strong alpha-adrenergic stimulator which also has had no medical use in urology (Boyarsky and Labay 1972), but has great theoretical use in the laboratory for identifying alpha-adrenergic receptors and the effect upon peristaltic activity of their stimul-ation (Weiss et al. 1978).

Adrenaline. Adrenaline is both an alpha- and a beta-adrenergic agonist. Since the effects of alpha and beta stimulation are opposite, the net effect may differ in the ureters of different species, or from one part of the ureter to the other (Weiss 1981b). Adrenaline can increase the amplitude and frequency of contrac-tion (Gruber 1930). Alpha blocking agents block the excitatory effect (Deane 1967) while a beta blocker such as propranolol can potentiate it (Vereecken 1973).

Isoproterenol (Isuprel). Isoproterenol is the classical prototype beta-adrenergic stimulator. It inhibits ureteric function, decreasing both amplitude and rate of peristalsis in vivo and in vitro (Boyarsky and Labay 1972; McLeod et al. 1973; Hannappel and Goldenhofen 1974). Due to its vigorous cardiovascular action, isoproterenol has had no place in the treatment of ureteric diseases.

Sympatholytic Agents

Phentolamine (Regitine). Phentolamine is an alpha-adrenergic blocking agent which can block the excitatory effect of catecholamines on the calices, renal pelvis and ureter, but has no demonstrable action on peristalsis. It has been tried by Peters and Eckstein (1975) in treating ureteric colic, after Kubacz and Catchpole (1972). In dogs, Peters and Eckstein noted dilatation of the intrinsically obstructed ureter and an increase in ureteric perfusate flow rate after its administration. They reported that 21 of 33 patients with renal colic were relieved by Regitine injection. This drug has not been in the first line of ureteric colic treatment, but could be considered for relief of pain and shortening the time of passage of a stone.

Phenoxybenzamine (Dibenzyline). Phenoxybenzamine is a long-acting alpha-adrenergic blocker. It takes longer to build a significant tissue level of this drug than of phentolamine. There is no clinical experience with this drug on the ureter.

Propranolol. Propranolol is a beta-adrenergic blocking agent. As is true for the alpha-adrenergic blockers, this beta blocker has no direct effect on intact dog and rat ureters (Kaplan et al. 1968; Boyarsky and Labay 1972). It abolishes the inhibitory effect of Isuprel and potentiates the contractile effect of noradrenaline and adrenaline (Weiss et al. 1970; Vereecken 1973). This drug has had no use in treating ureteric diseases.

Cholinergic Agents

Acetylcholine. There is no proven function yet for the cholinergic innervation of the ureter, although there are many cholinergic fibres and a few cholinergic cells and ganglion cells in the lowermost ureter (Elbadawi and Schenk 1969; Schulman 1975). However, acetylcholine can act on the ureter by releasing catecholamines from sympathetic ganglia and the adrenal gland. Hence, its action resembles that of noradrenaline in the intact organism, increasing ureteric peristaltic amplitude and frequency (Rose and Gillenwater 1974). This action is blocked by phentolamine (Rose and Gillenwater 1974). We have shown that bilateral adrenalectomy can prevent the action of acetylcholine on the ureter in the dog (Labay et al. 1968; Boyarsky and Labay 1972), which suggests that the source of catecholamine is the adrenal medulla as well as the sympathetic nerve endings, and provides further evidence for the indirect effect of acetylcholine on the ureter.

Methacholine (Mecholyl). Methacholine is a long-acting cholinergic agent.

There are controversial reports on its action on the ureter, some citing increased frequency and amplitude of ureteric peristalsis (Boatman et al. 1967) and others failing to observe such an action.

Bethanechol (Urecholine). Bethanechol has a prolonged cholinergic action of the muscarinic type. It increases ureteric peristalsis, an effect which is blocked by both atropine and phentolamine. Our experimental work (bilateral adrenalectomy in dogs: Labay et al. 1968) suggested strongly that its effect on ureteric peristalsis was through its adrenal secretagogic action. It has not been used in the treatment of ureteric diseases.

Anticholinergic Agents

Atropine. Atropine has an antimuscarinic action as an anticholinergic agent. It has no effect on ureteric peristalsis either in vivo or in vitro in many species including the human (Weinberg 1962). In general it inhibits the excitatory effect of cholinergic agents, physostigmine, adrenaline (in high concentration) and morphine. It is of no use in treating ureteric colic.

Propantheline (Pro-Banthine) and Methantheline (Banthine). Propantheline and methantheline are parasympathetic blocking agents with both antinicotinic and antimuscarinic actions. In the human they have no effect on ureteric peristalsis, even in large doses (Weinberg 1962; Montague and Straffon 1981). They may relax a previously contracted ureter, possibly by action on the preganglionic sympathetic system, and may distend a ureter as the result of inducing bladder retention. These anticholinergic drugs have been used together with analgesics to relieve ureteric colic, with considerable reported success (Montague and Straffon 1981). For example, the use of banthine as an intravenous injection (100–150 mg), together with an analgesic, was reported to be a very effective mode of treatment (Montague and Straffon 1981).

Non-steroidal Anti-inflammatory Agents

Indomethacin. Indomethacin, an anti-inflammatory agent, acts as a prostaglandin inhibitor. It decreases urine production and also has analgesic properties. In recent years there have been several reports on its use in the treatment of ureteric colic as shown by Marsala (1980). Holmlund and Sjödin (1978) carried out a double-blind study on the effect of 50 mg indomethacin given intravenously and found 76% of patients (31 of 41) had complete relief of pain as compared with 27% (7 of 26) in the controls. No side-effects were observed. They concluded that indomethacin in a concentration of 1 mg/kg decreases urine flow, and probably reduces oedema in the region of the stone.

Drugs which Show the Promise of Influencing Ureteric Activity

Ureteric physiology has produced large quantities of data which suggest that the ureter has its own unique physiology, is a very dynamic system sensitive to many classes of drugs (Weiss 1981), and contains many receptors. Ureteric epithelial function has never been explained. It behoves the astute urologist to remain abreast of basic developments in science, and to be alert for the clinical case that may benefit from a new agent which has first appeared on the market for use on another organ but can be adapted to the treatment of ureteric colic. Several such agents are mentioned here in order to make the urologist aware of their potential use, but no complete or authoritative review is intended. In this group of drugs we include the following:

Prostaglandins. PGE_1 can inhibit ureteric activity in vivo (Boyarsky et al. 1966) and in vitro by producing hyperpolarisation of the muscle membrane, and by sequestration of calcium ions at the inner side of the cell membrane. It also inhibits responses to electrical and mechanical stimulation. Conversely, $PGF_{2\alpha}$ increases peristaltic activity (Boyarsky and Labay 1969). PGE_2 is excreted by the renal medulla and improves renal blood flow and urine production, and may thereby stimulate ureteric peristalsis through its diuretic effect (Fulgraff and Brandenbusch 1974). With increasing clinical knowledge and experience, the prostaglandins may prove to have a useful role in treating ureteric disease.

Diphenhydramine (Benadryl) and Tripelennamine (Pyribenzamine). Diphenhydramine and tripelennamine act as antihistamines, and can inhibit the action of histamine competitively (Borgstedt et al. 1962). Some studies in dogs have shown an increase in ureteric peristalsis at certain dose levels (Sharkey et al. 1965) and an inhibitory action at others, consistent with competitive inhibition for the same receptor sites.

Histamine. Histamine has a direct action on smooth muscle, releasing potassium ions and depolarising the muscle cell membrane, and also releases catecholamines from the sympathetic nerve endings (Vereecken 1973). Histamine can cause contraction of the ureteric muscle, increasing the amplitude and frequency of peristalsis both in vivo and in vitro (Chen et al. 1957; Boyarsky and Labay 1967). The effect of histamine on the ureter differs from one species to another, being very active in dog, guinea-pig and pig but having no effect in rat and rabbit. It has been studied extensively in our laboratory and raises a host of interesting possibilities for research into drug mechanisms.

Serotonin. Serotonin has an excitatory effect on dog ureters in vitro, and increases both the frequency and amplitude of contractions (Boatman et al. 1967).

Metoclopramide (Pramine, Primperan). Metoclopramide is a procainamide derivative which acts on the smooth muscle of the ureter. Schelin (1979) described its use in the treatment of 4 patients with ureteric obstruction. It created rapid, vigorous peristalsis, with increased diuresis and markedly decreased hydronephrosis.

Glucagon. The hormone glucagon can inhibit ureteric peristalsis. It probably stimulates the production of cyclic AMP, thus causing muscle relaxation (Boyarsky and Labay 1978). Lowman et al. (1977) reported that glucagon caused ureteric relaxation in patients with ureteric calculi, reducing the pain in ureteric colic and producing rapid passage of stones from the ureter; others, however, have failed to confirm this.

Progesterone. During pregnancy this hormone may facilitate relaxation of the ureter, which is under compression by the gravid uterus. Its mode of action is most probably via antagonism of catecholamine action. Studies in vitro suggest that the ratio of beta- to alpha-adrenergic receptors in the ureter increases in pregnancy. We have been unable to confirm any primary action of progesterone on the dog ureter, and most workers doubt whether it has any significant effect on ureteric function (Boyarsky and Labay 1972). Perlow (1980) reported the prompt passage of stones in 2 patients after the administration of hydroxyprogesterone caproate (750 mg intramuscularly).

Oestrogens. Oestrogen has been reported to increase the amplitude and frequency of ureteric contractions, but we have not confirmed these reports in laboratory models, either in vivo or in vitro (Boyarsky and Labay 1972).

Silver Nitrate. Silver nitrate, as a locally applied diluted solution of 0.5%, has been tried in benign chronic bleeding with some success (Diamond et al. 1981). It has also been tried in the treatment of ureteritis cystica, with disappointing results. It is administered through a ureteric catheter or nephrostomy tube at a low-pressure drip for 10–30 minutes. Its effect is entirely destructive, like a chemical cautery, the aim being to denature protein, coagulate bleeding vessels or destroy tissue so as to halt a localised pathological process.

References

Boatman DL, Lewin ML, Culp DA, Flock RH (1967) Pharmacologic evaluation of ureteral smooth muscle. A technique for monitoring ureteral peristalsis. Invest Urol 4:509–520
Borgstedt HH (1960) Effects of some local anaesthetics, ganglion and NMJ-blockers on the electrically stimulated isolated dog ureter. Fed Proc 19:194
Borgstedt HH, Benjamin JA, Emmel VM (1962) The role of histamine in ureteral function. J Pharmacol Exp Ther 139:386–392
Boyarsky S, Labay P (1967) Histamine analog effect on the ureter. Invest Urol 4:351–365
Boyarsky S, Labay P (1969) Ureteral motility. Annu Rev Med 20:383–394
Boyarsky S, Labay P (1972) Methods. The physiology of ureteral peristalsis. Ureteral pharmacology. In: Boyarsky S (ed) Ureteral dynamics. Williams & Wilkins, Baltimore, Chaps. 1,2,5
Boyarsky S, Labay PC (1978) Glucagon, ureteral colic and ureteral peristalsis. Trans Am Assoc Genitourinary Surg 70:22–24
Boyarsky S, Labay P, Gerber C (1966) Prostaglandin inhibition of ureteral peristalsis. Invest Urol 4:9–11
Caine M (1981) Diseases of the ureter. In: Bergman H (ed) The ureter, 2nd ed. Springer-Verlag, Berlin Heidelberg New York, p 201

Chen PS, Emmel VM, Benjamin JA, Distefano V (1957) Studies on the isolated dog ureter. The pharmacological action of histamine, levartrenol, and antihistaminics. Arch Int Pharmacodyn 110:131–141

Davis JE, Hagedroon JP, Bergmann LL (1981) Anatomy and ultrastructure of the ureter. In: Bergman H (ed) The ureter, 2nd ed. Springer-Verlag, Berlin Heidelberg New York, pp 60–61

Deane RF (1967) Functional studies of the ureter: its behavior in the domestic pig as recorded by the technique of Trendelenburg. Br J Urol 39:31–37

Diamond DA, Jeffs RD, Marshall FF (1981) Control of prolonged benign renal hematuria by silver nitrate instillation. Urology 18:337–341

Elbadawi A, Schenk EA (1969) Innervation of the abdominopelvic ureter in the cat. Am J Anat 126:103–119

Elliott JP, Evans JW, Gordon JO, Platt LO (1979) Butorphanol and meperidine compared in patients with acute ureteral colic. J Urol 122:455–457

Fulgraff G, Brandenbusch G (1974) Comparison of the effects of prostaglandins A_1, E_2 and F_2 on kidney function in dogs. Pflügers Arch 349:9–17

Gardner B, Whitaker RH (1981) The use of danazol for ureteral obstruction caused by endometriosis. J Urol 125:117–118

Gruber CM (1928) The effect of morphine and papaverine upon the peristaltic and antiperistaltic contraction of the ureter. J Pharmacol Exp Ther 33:191–199

Gruber CM (1930) The effect of epinephrine upon the rate of contraction and upon the conduction time of peristalsis and antiperistalsis in excised ureters. J Pharmacol Exp Ther 39:449–456

Hallwachs O, Baar R (1972) Combined tuberculostatic and corticoid therapy of tuberculous ureteral stricture. Med Welt 23(5):174–176 (in German)

Hannappel J, Goldenhofen K (1974) The effect of catecholamines on ureteral peristalsis in different species (dog, guinea pig, and rat). Pflügers Arch 350:55–68

Holmlund D (1968) Ureteral stones. An experimental and clinical study of the mechanism of the passage and arrest of ureteral stones. Scand J Urol Nephrol [Suppl] 1

Holmlund D, Hassler O (1965) A method of studying the ureteral reaction to artificial concrements. Acta Chir Scand 130:335–343

Holmlund D, Sjödin JG (1978) Treatment of ureteral colic with intravenous indomethacin. J Urol 120:676–677

Kaplan N, Elkin M, Sharkey J (1968) Ureteral peristalsis and the autonomic nervous system. Invest Urol 5:468–482

Kim HL, Labay PC, Boyarsky S, Glenn JF (1970) An experimental model of ureteral colic. J Urol 104:390–394

Kinn AC, Boreus LO, Nergardh A (1982) Effects of narcotic analgesics, especially pethidine and nor-pethidine on renal pelvis smooth muscles in patients with hydronephrosis. Eur J Clin Pharmacol 22:407–410

Kubacz GJ, Catchpole BN (1972) The role of adrenergic blockade in the treatment of ureteral colic. J Urol 107:949–951

Labay PC, Boyarsky S, Herlong JH (1968) Relation of adrenal to ureteral function. Fed Proc 27:444 (no. 1276)

Lowman RM et al. (1977) Glucagon (letter to the editor). J Urol 118:128

McLeod DG, Reynolds DG, Swan KG (1973) Adrenergic mechanisms in the canine ureter. Am J Physiol 224:1054–1058

Malin JM Jr, Boyarsky S, Labay P, Gerber C (1968) In vitro isometric studies of ureteral smooth muscle. J Urol 99:396–398

Malin JM Jr, Deane RF, Boyarsky S (1970) Characterisation of adrenergic receptors in human ureter. Br J Urol 42:171–174

Marsala F (1980) Treatment of ureteral and biliary pain with an injectable salt of indomethacin. Pharmatherapeutica 2(6):357–362

Montague DK, Straffon RA (1981) Ureteral calculi. In: Bergman H (ed) The ureter, 2nd ed. Springer-Verlag, Berlin Heidelberg New York, p 261

Olshwang D, Shapiro A, Perlberg S, Magora F (1984) The effect of epidural morphine on ureteral colic and spasm of the bladder. Pain 18:97–101

Perlow DL (1980) The use of progesterone for ureteral stone: a preliminary report. J Urol 124:715–716

Peters HJ, Eckstein W (1975) Possible pharmacological means of treating renal colic. Urol Res 3:55–59

Risholm L (1954) Studies on renal colic and its treatment by posterior splanchnic block. Acta Chir Scand [Suppl] 184:1–64

Rose JG, Gillenwater JY (1974) The effect of adrenergic and cholinergic agents and their blockers upon ureteral activity. Invest Urol 11:439–451

Schelin S (1979) Observations on the effect of metoclopramide (Primperan) on human ureter. A preliminary communication. Scand J Urol Nephrol 13:79–82

Schulman CC (1975) Ultrastructural evidence for adrenergic and cholinergic innervation of the human ureter. J Urol 113:765–771

Sharkey J, Boyarsky S, Catacutan-Labay P, Martinez J (1965) The in vivo effects of histamine and benadryl on the peristalsis of the canine ureter and plasma potassium levels. Invest Urol 2:417–427

Shiratori T, Kinoshita H (1961) Electromyographic studies on urinary tract. II. Electromyographic study on the genesis of peristaltic movement of the dog's ureter. Tohoku J Exp Med 73:103–117

Sternberg JJ, Bracken BR, Handel PB, Johnson DE (1977) Combination chemotherapy (CISCA) for advanced urinary tract carcinoma. JAMA 238:2282–2287

Struthers NW (1973) An experimental model for evaluating drug effects on the ureter. Br J Urol 45:23–27

Vereecken RL (1973) Dynamic aspects of urine transport in the ureter. Acco, Louvain

Weinberg SR (1962) Application of physiologic principles to surgery of the ureter. Am J Surg 103:549–554

Weiss RM (1981a) Effects of drugs on the ureter. In: Bergman H (ed) The ureter, 2nd ed. Springer-Verlag, Berlin Heidelberg New York, pp 138, 139

Weiss RM (1981b) Effects of drugs on the ureters. In: Bergman H (ed) The ureter, 2nd ed. Springer-Verlag, Berlin Heidelberg New York, p 143

Weiss RM, Bassett AL, Hoffman BF (1970) Effect of ouabain on contractility of the isolated ureter. Invest Urol 8:161–169

Yagoda A, Watson RC, Kemeny N, Barzell WE, Grabstald H, Whitmore WF Jr (1978) Diaminedichloride platinum II and cyclophosphamide in the treatment of advanced urothelial cancer. Cancer 41:2121–2130

Chapter 5

Pharmacological Management of the Neuropathic Bladder and Urethra

Ananias C. Diokno and L. Paul Sonda

The demand upon physicians to treat a growing number of patients with neuro-pathic bladder and urethra can be traced to a variety of reasons. The improved emergency services and intensive care provided for trauma victims have resulted in an increased survival of patients, many of whom have spinal cord and peripheral nerve injury. Additionally, the increased use of newer diagnostic equipment and an increased index of suspicion for neuropathic bladder disorders have improved our ability to recognise these problems. Extensive dissemination of new information pertaining to neurogenic bladder and sphincter dysfunctions has thrust the problem into a more prominent position in modern medical practice.

In earlier years, the diagnosis of neuropathic bladder usually resulted in lifelong catheter drainage or a urinary diversion. Just as the recognition of neurogenic bladder dysfunction has increased, so has knowledge regarding treatment. Newer therapy has improved the outlook for these patients by offering more choices. Specific therapy is now available which can achieve better results. One of the most important advances is in the pharmacological management of neurogenic bladder and sphincter dysfunction.

Neural Control of Micturition

The urinary bladder, bladder neck and external sphincter are under the control of the cerebrospinal nervous system. The cerebral centre for micturition is believed to be located in the frontal lobe of the brain. From the frontal cortex, fibres descend into the detrusor motor nucleus located in the brain stem (Raz and Bradley 1979). From this nucleus, fibres descend within the spinal cord as the cortico-regulatory tract and synapse with the neurons located in the sacral segments 2, 3 and 4. This is considered to be the spinal cord centre for micturition (Lapides and Diokno 1976). These sacral cord segments are located at about the bony level of thoracic 12 to lumbar 1 vertebral bodies. From these sacral segments originate two important nerves: the pelvic nerve, a parasympathetic nerve that originates in the lateral horn cells and supplies motor impulses to the bladder and urethra, and the pudendal nerve, a somatic nerve that originates in the ventral horn cells and innervates the external sphincter. The activity of these two nerves is synchronised under normal conditions. Thus, increased activity of the pelvic nerve is associated with inhibition of pudendal nerve activity; and conversely, increased activity of the pudendal nerve is associated with reduced activity of the pelvic nerve.

The sympathetic nerve supply to the bladder and internal sphincter is through the presacral nerve, which originates from the lower thoracic and upper lumbar spinal cord segments via the hypogastric ganglia. There are two distinct adrenergic receptors in the bladder and urethra. The body of the bladder above the trigone is rich in beta receptors, while the trigone and the proximal or posterior urethra are rich in alpha receptors. Stimulation of the beta receptors produces relaxation of the detrusor smooth muscle; alpha receptor activation causes increase in the tone of the smooth muscle (Awad et al. 1974).

The neurotransmitters, chemical substances that transmit impulses from the nerve ending to the effector site or between one nerve ending and another neuron, are acetylcholine and noradrenaline. Acetylcholine is released at the parasympathetic preganglionic and postganglionic, the sympathetic preganglionic, and the somatic nerve endings. Noradrenaline is released at the sympathetic postganglionic fibres.

The exteroceptive and proprioceptive sensations of the bladder are transmitted through the afferents of both the pelvic and presacral nerves, reaching the higher centres through the lateral spinothalamic tract and the posterior column respectively. The pudendal nerve serves as the afferent tract for the sensation coming from the external genitalia and the perineum.

Mechanism of Normal Micturition

In babies and children up to the age of 2 to 3, voiding is accomplished reflexly. Afferent impulses coming from the bladder wall undergoing distension are perceived by the detrusor sensory neurons. These neurons activate the brain stem/sacral reflex arc, eventually sending impulses back to the bladder, causing the detrusor to produce a sustained contraction. Before the recorded rise in intravesical pressure, the peri-urethral striated muscle, or the external sphincter, becomes totally relaxed (Fig. 5.1). As the detrusor contracts, the bladder neck opens. Urine flow generally starts when a detrusor pressure of 30 cm of water or more is achieved. Flow is continuous, with a maximum flow rate of 25 ml per second or greater. In older children and adults, voiding is initiated voluntarily through the described tracts originating from the cerebral cortex. Normally, micturition can be stopped at any moment by the instantaneous action of the external sphincter upon the urethra and by the slower-acting inhibition of detrusor contraction.

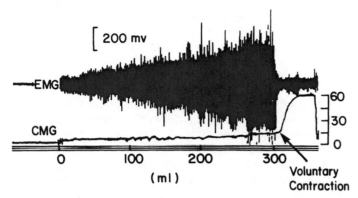

Fig. 5.1. Combined cystometry and needle sphincter electromyography showing normal detrusor and sphincter function. The peri-urethral striated muscle relaxes just prior to the onset of voluntary detrusor contraction.

Definition and Types of Neuropathic Bladder and Urethra

Neurogenic bladder and sphincter dysfunctions are the result of injury to or disease of the neuronal control of the lower urinary tract. The disturbance can be anywhere from the cerebral cortex to the peripheral nerves. The terms 'neuropathic bladder' or 'neurogenic bladder' do not represent a single entity but encompass a constellation of lower urinary tract problems depending upon several factors. These factors include the site and extent of the lesion, the duration of the neurological disturbance and previous treatment of the condition.

There are numerous ways to categorise neuropathic disturbances of the bladder and sphincter. From the point of view of understanding the neurological lesions and the resultant bladder dysfunction, the classification of Lapides has been useful (Lapides and Diokno 1976). This classification has the distinct advantage of grossly localising the site of neurological disturbance. The disadvantage is a relative inability to classify mixed and incomplete lesions where the urological dysfunction does not fit neatly into any of the categories of neurogenic bladder.

The five types of neuropathic bladder are as follows:

1) *Uninhibited neurogenic bladder* is due to lesions involving the cortico-regulatory tract anywhere along the cerebrospinal axis above sacral segments 2–4. It is believed that the lesions involve the inhibitory fibres of the cortico-regulatory tract. These patients are unable to control their sudden detrusor contractions and resultant urge to void, although they can initiate voiding voluntarily. They have urinary frequency, urgency, urge incontinence and enuresis. The condition is frequently seen in patients with previous cerebrovascular accidents and incomplete spinal cord injury. It should also be suspected

in a patient who 'completely recovered' from spinal cord injury but experiences the above bladder symptomatology. The manifestations of an uninhibited bladder usually appear a few weeks after the cerebral or spinal lesion has stabilised. Some patients with multiple sclerosis may present with an uninhibited bladder. However, the specific bladder and sphincter dysfunction may be transient and may evolve to another type, depending upon the location of the plaques. Certain patients with uninhibited neurogenic bladder may exhibit no history or physical findings suggesting neurological injury or disease. Cystometry will document the presence of uninhibited bladder contractions, normal bladder sensation and ability to initiate voluntary detrusor contraction (Fig.5.2).

2) *Reflex neurogenic bladder* is due to complete injury or extensive disease of the spinal cord above sacral segments 2–4. The most common clinical conditions associated with reflex neurogenic bladder are paraplegia and quadriplegia after the recovery from the period of spinal shock. Patients with advanced multiple sclerosis may also develop this bladder abnormality. These patients lack exteroceptive and proprioceptive sensation. Voiding is totally involuntary, and therefore they are incontinent of urine. Cystometry will demonstrate the presence of uninhibited contractions, without voluntary control of micturition and with absent bladder sensation (Fig. 5.3).

3) *Motor paralytic bladder* is characterised by lesions involving the peripheral motor fibres to the detrusor or the detrusor motor neurons located in the sacral spinal cord segments. Exteroceptive and proprioceptive sensations are preserved, so that these patients are uncomfortable as the result of bladder distension but are unable to empty their bladders due to the absence of any detrusor contractions. Excellent examples are patients after radical pelvic surgery such as radical hysterectomy and abdomino-perineal resections of the rectosigmoid, severe pelvic fracture, or Landry–Guillain-Barré disease. Spinal stenosis occurring in the lumbar spine area can also produce a motor paralytic bladder. Cystometry will demonstrate an areflexic cystometrograph, normal bladder sensation, and a positive bethanechol supersensitivity test.

The bethanechol supersensitivity test was devised by Lapides and co-workers in 1962. It was based on the denervation supersensitivity phenomenon (Cannon and Rosenbleuth 1949) and has the express purpose of diagnosing neurogenic bladder dysfunction. Such a test is indicated whenever a neurogenic cause is suspected for the patient's voiding complaints, such as sensory deficits in the bladder and/or perineum, significant residual urine (> 50 ml), and obstructive lower urinary tract symptoms without demonstrable anatomical obstruction. Positive results should prompt more extensive neurological testing. Spinal cord tumours, herniated discs and other neurological disorders masquerading as chronic, simple urinary tract disturbances can be identified with the aid of this valuable test.

The test is performed by means of a standard retrograde cystometry using either gas or water as the infusing medium. The usual flow rate is 100 ml/minute. After obtaining the baseline cystometrograph, 2.5 mg of bethanechol chloride is given subcutaneously. Cystometry is repeated at 20 minutes after the administration of the test dose, and the intravesical pressures at 100 ml of bladder capacity before and after the bethanechol dose are compared. If the increase in intravesical pressure is less than 20 cm of water, the test is negative, suggesting no evidence of significant denervation in the sacral spinal cord or peripheral nerves. If the pressure rise is greater than 20 cm, the test is considered

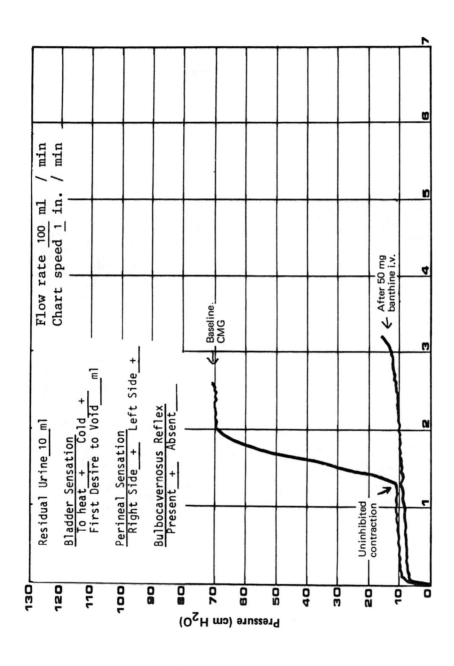

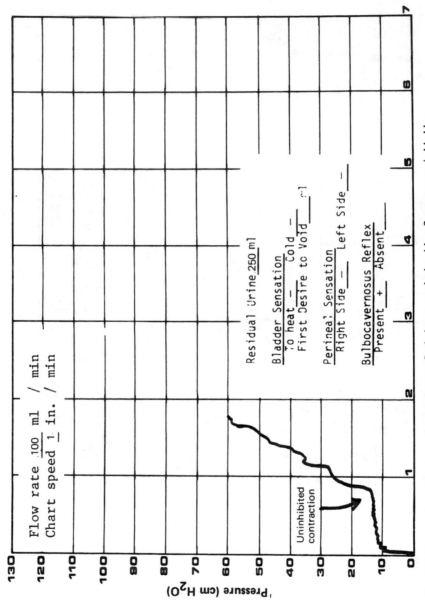

Fig. 5.3. Cystometrograph demonstrating hyperreflexia in a paraplegic with reflex neurogenic bladder.

positive and suggests significant denervation. In general, a positive response is characterised by a marked increase in pressure exceeding the minimum of 20 cm of water. False positives have been observed in patients with azotaemia. Our laboratory study using dogs has shown that the supersensitive response of the detrusor develops within 1–3 weeks after bilateral denervation. Most of the unilaterally denervated bladders (10/11 dogs) did not develop the supersensitivity response. This finding (Diokno et al. 1975) suggests that extensive denervation is required to provoke a positive test. Thus, the test may be falsely negative in situations where only partial nerve damage has occurred.

4) *Autonomous neurogenic bladder* results from a total destruction of sacral segments 2–4 or extensive injury to both motor and sensory nerve supply to the bladder. Spinal cord tumours and trauma producing complete injury to sacral segments 2–4 or lower can result in this type of bladder dysfunction. The spinal shock stage seen during the early phase of spinal cord injury or the acute stage of multiple sclerosis also produces an autonomous type of neurogenic bladder. The abnormality is usually transient and can evolve into a totally different pattern of bladder dysfunction, depending upon recovery of the spinal cord from the injury or the disease. These patients are unable to void voluntarily or to perceive bladder sensation or distension. They may also have overflow urinary incontinence or even stress incontinence depending upon the state of external sphincter function. Cystometry will demonstrate an areflexic bladder with no sensation and a positive bethanechol supersensitivity test (Fig. 5.4). The test will be negative during the spinal shock phase.

5) *Sensory paralytic bladder* is the result of lesions involving the afferent nerve tracts innervating the bladder as well as the fibres coursing the posterior column or the lateral spinothalamic tracts. This type of bladder is usually seen in patients with tabes dorsalis, syringomyelia, or occasionally diabetes. These patients are infrequent voiders due to absent or poor bladder perception. The bladder condition is rarely discovered until the occurrence of urinary retention or urinary tract infection. Cystometry will demonstrate a large-capacity bladder without any uninhibited contractions. Voluntary detrusor contractions may or may not be present, depending upon the degree of detrusor tonicity. The bethanechol supersensitivity test is positive.

Types of Neuropathic Sphincter

External sphincter dysfunction secondary to a neurogenic cause can be sub-divided into two categories (Diokno et al. 1974). The first category is caused by the state of external sphincter innervation. Sphincter denervation is usually due to injury to or disease of either the pudendal motor neurons at the anterior horn of sacral segments 2–4, or the pudendal nerves themselves. The denervation can be partial or complete. A partially denervated external sphincter may manifest only mild stress incontinence; progressive amounts of denervation will produce more significant degrees of incontinence. Sphincter denervation is usually associated with a motor paralytic or autonomous neurogenic bladder, but can occur independently (Fig. 5.5). Needle electromyography of the peri-

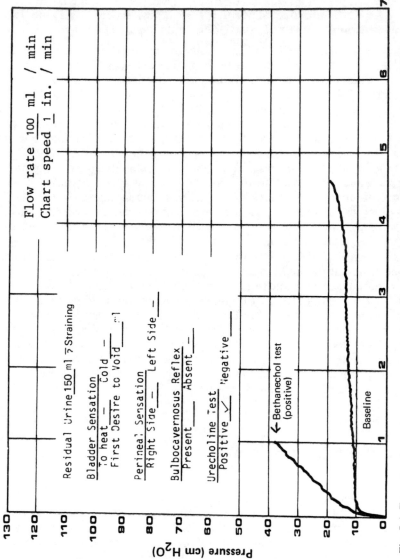

Fig. 5.4. Example of an autonomous neurogenic bladder. Note the positive bethanechol supersensitivity test.

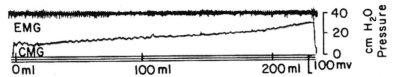

Fig. 5.5. Combined cystometry and needle sphincter electromyography showing an areflexic bladder and severely denervated striated sphincter.

urethral striated muscle will demonstrate the presence of denervation potentials such as positive waves and fibrillations, with a decrease or even absence of normal motor units (Fig. 5.6).

The second category is caused by the state of function of the innervated external sphincter. It should first be determined whether striated sphincter activity is under voluntary control or responds involuntarily. Regardless of which is the case, the degree to which the striated sphincter is coordinated or uncoordinated with the detrusor contraction must be assessed. Most of the patients with an uninhibited neurogenic bladder have voluntary control and coordination of the sphincter.

When testing a patient with hyperreflexia, an attempt should be made to distinguish a true involuntary detrusor sphincter dyssynergia from a false or voluntary dyssynergia. In a patient with hyperreflexia the tendency is to control voiding by contracting the peri-urethral striated muscle. After one or two episodes of hyperreflexia the patient should be instructed to overcome the involuntary sphincter contraction by voluntary voiding. At this point a patient with normal external sphincter control should be able to relax the peri-urethral striated muscle in conjunction with a detrusor contraction (Fig. 5.7). Approximately two-thirds of all paraplegics with reflex bladders have uncoordinated or dyssynergic sphincters (Fig. 5.8) (Perlow and Diokno 1980). Cystometry combined with electromyography (Diokno et al. 1974), or detrusor pressure flow/electromyographic studies will diagnose the presence of sphincter dyssynergia with detrusor function (Yalla et al. 1976).

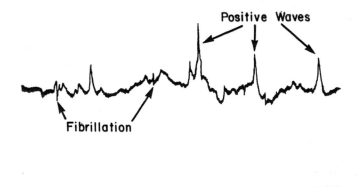

Fig. 5.6. Needle electromyography of the peri-urethral striated muscle showing fibrillations and positive waves suggestive of denervation.

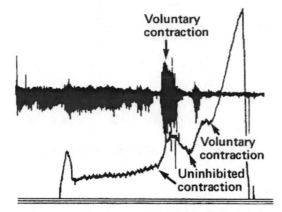

Fig. 5.7. Combined cystometry and sphincter electromyography in an incontinent patient who had a cerebrovascular accident. The tracings show involuntary detrusor contractions and voluntary sphincter hyperactivity followed by voluntary voiding with appropriate sphincter relaxation.

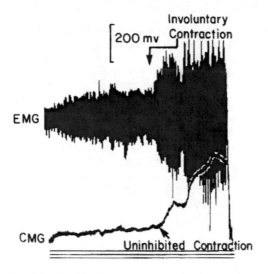

Fig. 5.8. Combined cystometry and needle sphincter electromyography in a paraplegic patient showing uninhibited contraction and hyperactivity of the peri-urethral striated muscle (uncoordinated sphincter).

Gosling and co-workers (1981) have recently described a rhabdosphincter or urethral musculature that is histologically, histochemically and electron microscopically different from the levator ani and the peri-urethral striated muscle. In its present state, clinical electromyography cannot distinguish the difference between such muscles.

The lack of reliable electromyography for smooth muscle has made it impossible to diagnose urethral smooth muscle denervation directly. The diagnosis must be inferred from the history of previous nerve injury or disease. Alpha-adrenergic supersensitivity testing of the denervated smooth muscle of the urethra has been suggested and may shed more light on the evaluation of the internal sphincter (Koyanagi and Tsuji 1978). Internal sphincter dyssynergia can be diagnosed by administering an alpha blocker, phentolamine, and then measuring the change in urine flow using a flowmeter or observing changes in the bladder neck using radiographic means (Krane and Olsson 1973). Simultaneous pressure–flow studies with fluoroscopy and urethral pressure monitoring can evaluate urethral smooth muscle function more specifically.

General Principles of Therapy

The goals of therapy for patients with a neuropathic bladder and sphincter are twofold. The first major objective is to preserve renal function. Preventing overdistension and high bladder pressure by frequent or continuous low-pressure bladder emptying can help accomplish this goal, as also can avoidance of urinary tract infection and urolithiasis. The second, equally important objective is to help these patients return to social acceptability. This can be accomplished by controlling urinary incontinence, and by management of any appliances or devices patients may be using.

Pharmacotherapy of Neuropathic Bladder and Urethra

The concept of using drugs in the treatment of bladder dysfunction is not new. However, newer drugs have become available which broaden the treatment options. When using pharmacological agents, a clear understanding of the underlying pathophysiological disturbance in the bladder and/or urethra will increase the chances of achieving the optimal result. Thus, an adequate evaluation must be performed before embarking on a treatment plan. The major problems are urinary retention and urinary incontinence, which in many cases may coexist. In patients with urinary incontinence, the practitioner must know the cause of the incontinence to treat the patient effectively. Often, simple urodynamic tests will identify the patient with detrusor hyperreflexia as opposed to urethral sphincter dysfunction, or a combination of the two.

A major guideline in choosing a pharmacological agent is to establish the goal of therapy. If the goal is to control urinary incontinence, then the choice is either to increase bladder capacity using an anticholinergic/antispasmodic preparation, or to increase urethral resistance using an alpha-adrenergic agent. Sometimes both options are pursued by employing a combination of the two agents. If the goal is to facilitate emptying, then the choices include the use of a cholinergic agent, an alpha-adrenergic blocker, a skeletal muscle relaxant, or a combination of the three agents. The pharmacological agents have specific target sites, and a combination of therapeutic modalities may be necessary in order to obtain the desired goal.

Drugs That Increase Bladder Capacity: Anticholinergic/Antispasmodic Agents (Table 5.1)

Drugs that help to increase bladder capacity by inhibiting uncontrolled detrusor contractions fall into two groups. One group is the anticholinergics, which can be subdivided into (1) belladonna alkaloids, (2) quaternary ammonium derivatives of the belladonna alkaloids, and (3) synthetic substitutes. Anticholinergic agents block the effects of acetylcholine at the postganglionic cholinergic endings (Fig. 5.2).

Table 5.1. Anticholinergic/antispasmodic agents

Drug	Preparation	Dosage[a]
Belladonna, tincture	40 drops/ml (0.3 mg atropine)	15–40 drops q.i.d. Paediatric: 8–20 drops t.i.d.–q.i.d.
Methscopolamine	2.5 mg tablet	2.5 mg t.i.d.
Propantheline	7.5 and 15 mg tablets	15–30 mg q.i.d. Paediatric: 7.5–15 mg q.i.d.
Oxybutynin	5 mg/5 ml 5 mg tablet	5–10 mg t.i.d.–q.i.d. Paediatric: 5 mg b.i.d.–t.i.d.
Dicyclomine	10 mg capsule 20 mg tablet 10 mg/5 ml	20 mg t.i.d.–q.i.d.

[a] Adult dosage unless otherwise specified. b.i.d., twice a day; t.i.d., three times a day; q.i.d., four times a day.

The second group comprises those preparations showing a combination of anticholinergic and antispasmodic effects, as exemplified by oxybutynin chloride and dicyclomine chloride. These drugs are indicated in patients with uninhibited bladder contractions to prevent urinary frequency, urgency, enuresis, and urge or precipitate urinary incontinence. Vinson and Diokno (1976) reported an 81% (49 of 60) success rate with the use of anticholinergic agents in controlling the symptoms of adult patients with uninhibited neurogenic bladders. Koff et al. (1979) have reported improvement of symptoms in 83% of 36 incontinent paediatric patients treated with a detrusor relaxant to control the uninhibited detrusor contractions causing urinary incontinence. The drug also reduced or eliminated daytime frequency, urgency and precipitate micturition.

Tincture of belladonna, an extract of belladonna leaves, works by virtue of its atropine content. It is used mainly in children or adults who cannot take solid preparations of an anticholinergic agent. The usual children's dose is 8–20 drops mixed in juice or milk and taken three or four times a day. The patient is generally started on a low dose, which is gradually increased until the desired effect is achieved with a minimum of side-effects. The usual adult dose is 40 drops or 1 ml, which is equivalent to 0.3 mg of atropine. The side-effects are the usual antimuscarinic effects, such as dryness of the mucous membrane, constipation, pupillary dilation, flushing and heat intolerance.

A representative of the quaternary ammonium derivatives of belladonna alkaloids is methscopolamine bromide (Pamine). It is available in 2.5 mg tablets which are taken three times a day; it is longer-acting, with no central action, but is poorly absorbed and less potent than atropine.

One of the most widely used anticholinergics is the synthetic quaternary ammonium compound represented by propantheline and methantheline (Finkbeiner and Bissada 1980). Its onset of action is 30 minutes after oral administration, and its duration of action is approximately 4 hours (Kieswetter and Popper 1972). The adult dosage of propantheline (Pro-Banthine) is 15 mg orally four times a day, which can be raised to 30 mg orally four times a day if needed. The usual children's dosage is 7.5 mg orally four times a day.

Among the synthetic anticholinergic/antispasmodic preparations, oxybutynin chloride is one of the most commonly used medications. Its effect lasts 8–10 hours (Diokno and Lapides 1972; Thompson and Lauvetz 1976). The usual dosage is 5 mg orally twice or three times a day for children and three times a day for adults. Syrup of Ditropan is available in 5 mg/5 ml dose. Its side-effects are similar to those of other anticholinergic preparations.

Another anticholinergic/antispasmodic preparation is dicyclomine chloride (Awad et al. 1977; Fischer et al. 1978). The usual dosage is 20 mg orally three times a day. The adverse reactions are similar to those of other antimuscarinic drugs.

The practising physician will have in his pharmacopoeia a variety of anticholinergic/antispasmodic agents from which to choose. In our experience, not all 'bladder relaxants' work equally well, nor do they produce the same intensity of side-effects. While a patient may be only partially responsive to, or complain of intolerable side-effects with, one medication, a similar preparation may be 'perfect' for that same patient. In general, we first give children a liquid preparation such as tincture of belladonna or syrup of oxybutynin, while adults start with either a synthetic anticholinergic such as propantheline or an anticholinergic/antispasmodic agent such as oxybutynin. We then use other anticholinergics as substitutes if the initial preparation fails to provide the expected result.

Drugs That Increase Sphincter Resistance: Sympathomimetic Agents (Table 5.2)

Sympathomimetic drugs used in urological practice are aimed at increasing sphincter resistance in patients with a mild to moderate degree of stress incontinence of both neurogenic and non-neurogenic origin. Neurogenic aetiologies include paralysis of the external and/or internal sphincter musculature. The alpha-adrenergic agents work by increasing the tone of the urethral smooth muscle by activating the alpha-adrenergic receptors; they have no effect on the skeletal musculature. Representative drugs in this category are ephedrine and

Table 5.2. Sympathomimetic agents

Drug	Preparation	Dosage[a]
Ephedrine	25 mg and 50 mg tablets and capsules	25–50 mg t.i.d.–q.i.d. Paediatric: 11–25 mg t.i.d.–q.i.d.
Phenylpropanolamine	25 and 50 mg tablets	50–100 mg b.i.d.

[a] Adult dosage unless otherwise specified. b.i.d., twice a day; t.i.d., three times a day; q.i.d., four times a day.

phenylpropanolamine. These drugs are contraindicated in patients with hypertension and thyroid disease.

Ephedrine, although occurring naturally in various plants, is now synthetically prepared. It has both alpha and beta receptor stimulating properties. In addition to its direct effect on the receptors, it has the ability to release noradrenaline from storage sites in the sympathetic nerves. Ephedrine is available as a 25 mg or 50 mg tablet or capsule. It also comes in the form of 4 mg/ml syrup. The dosage ranges from 44 mg daily to 200 mg daily in four divided doses. The common side-effects of this drug include hypertension, palpitation and insomnia. In a series of 38 patients with urinary incontinence from neurogenic and non-neurogenic causes, Diokno and Taub (1975) were able to achieve a good to excellent control in 27 patients (71%). They found ephedrine to be helpful when the incontinence was mild to moderate in degree, and ineffective in severe cases.

Phenylpropanolamine hydrochloride has similar pharmacological effects to those of ephedrine, except that it causes less central nervous stimulation (Awad et al. 1978). The drug is available in 25 mg or 50 mg capsules and in an elixir of 4 mg/ml. The usual adult dosage is 50–100 mg twice daily. It also comes as an ingredient in Ornade, which can be used as an oral preparation twice a day (Stewart et al. 1976). Each Ornade spansule contains 75 mg of phenylpropanolamine.

Beta blockers have been suggested as another type of drug for increasing urethral resistance; their action is indirect in that the effect of alpha-adrenergic receptors is potentiated once the beta receptor is blocked. This group has not been explored to any great extent, most probably because of the cardiovascular side-effects (Khanna 1976).

Drugs That Facilitate Bladder Emptying

Urinary retention, of either the complete or incomplete variety, may be due to an acontractile detrusor, increased outlet resistance, or both. The detrusor failure can be the result of detrusor denervation or hypotonicity. Cholinergic agents may improve bladder contractility. Outlet obstructions may be anatomical, as in cases of prostatism or urethral strictures, or functional, as the detrusor sphincter dyssynergia seen in many paraplegics. Cases of detrusor/internal sphincter dyssynergia may also be a cause of incomplete bladder emptying. Skeletal muscle relaxants have been used to treat detrusor sphincter dyssynergia. For internal sphincter dyssynergia, an alpha blocker has been recommended.

Cholinergic Agents (Table 5.3)

For detrusor failure due to partial paralysis or in suprasacral lesions where the detrusor contractions are weak, bethanechol chloride has been useful. The drug should never be used in patients with dyssynergia unless sphincterotomy has been performed or sphincter relaxant preparations are concomitantly administered.

Bethanechol chloride is a choline ester that acts directly on the effector cells. It is different from acetylcholine in that it is resistant to hydrolysis by

Table 5.3. Cholinergic agents

Drug	Preparation	Dosage[a]
Bethanechol	5 mg ampule	2.5–7.5 mg subcutaneously every 4–6 hours
	5, 10, 25 and 50 mg tablets	25–50 mg t.i.d.–q.i.d.

[a] Adult dosage. t.i.d., three times a day; q.i.d., four times a day.

cholinesterase. In patients with partial motor paralytic bladders who are able to void incompletely, with a poor stream and high residual volume but without anatomical or functional obstruction, bethanechol can improve the flow and decrease residual urine (Fig. 5.9). Treatment is lifelong unless the neurological lesion is corrected and bladder innervation is recovered. In patients with decompensation or hypotonicity due to sensory paralytic bladder, bethanechol has been used effectively to rehabilitate the bladder. The parenteral preparation is used initially; if successful, this is altered to an oral preparation. It is possible to taper the dose and even discontinue the drug altogether in some cases. In hyperreflexic bladders, bethanechol can be used to facilitate emptying when the reflex contractions are weak and inefficient, as long as the external sphincter is coordinated. It is also helpful in achieving complete bladder emptying in dyssynergic patients following successful sphincterotomy. In certain cases, the detrusor contractions are weak and unsustained, and unable to empty the bladder in spite of successful sphincterotomy (Diokno and Koppenhoefer 1976; Sonda et al. 1979). Sporer et al. (1978) have found in a series of 14 patients with high spinal cord lesions and postural detrusor external sphincter dyssynergia, that a combination of bethanechol chloride and dantrolene is the most logical pharmacological approach. They recommended a dosage of 150 mg of bethanechol orally per day and up to 300 mg of dantrolene orally per day.

The usual adult dosage is 25–50 mg orally three or four times a day. The usual parenteral dosage is 5 mg subcutaneously every 4–6 hours for 2 or 3 days. On occasion, 7.5 mg is the starting parenteral dose. This is gradually tapered by 2.5 mg until it is discontinued or converted to the oral dose. The common side-effects include sweating, nausea, abdominal cramps and salivation. Patients often must tolerate side-effects during initial parenteral therapy in order to achieve success. Severe side-effects can be counteracted by atropine.

Recent reports of the use of prostaglandin $F_{2\alpha}$ in patients with neurogenic bladder dysfunction showed that the drug given intravesically produces contractions that can induce voiding in patients with suprasacral lesions but not in patients with complete denervation, detrusor sphincter dyssynergia, or spinal shock bladder (Vaidyanathan et al. 1981). To date this drug remains experimental.

Skeletal Muscle Relaxants (Table 5.4)

Skeletal muscle relaxants can be grouped according to their site of action. The centrally acting drugs are the benzodiazepines, represented by diazepam (Valium) and baclofen (Lioresal). Diazepam's skeletal muscle relaxant effect, if any, is probably mediated by its central depressant action on the spinal reflex via the brain stem reticular system. Its effectiveness may be totally dependent on its anxiolytic property, a reason why this drug appears to be more effective

a

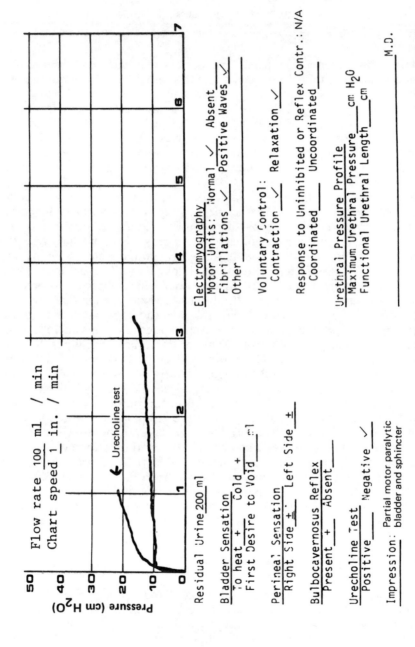

Fig. 5.9. a Cystometrograph of a young man who sustained an incomplete motor and sensory lesion at right L4 and left S1 secondary to a gunshot wound. The combined study showed an areflexic bladder, partial sphincter denervation and incomplete bladder emptying. The impression was an incomplete motor paralytic and sensory bladder and sphincter dysfunction.

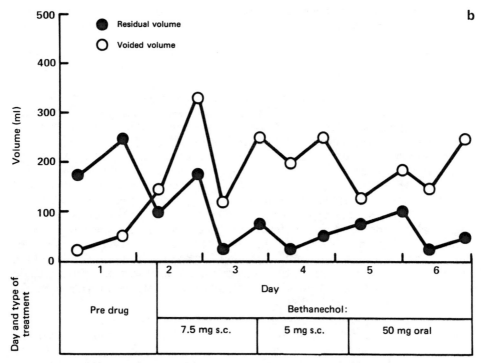

Fig. 5.9. b Same patient as in **a**. Voiding pattern before and after bethanechol therapy, showing recovery of bladder function.

for non-neurogenic detrusor dyssynergia (Smey et al. 1978). The usual adult dosage is 5 mg three or four times a day. The children's dosage is 0.2–0.4 mg/kg three or four times a day. The common side-effects are related to central nervous depression, drowsiness and ataxia.

Baclofen works by reducing polysynaptic reflex activity in the spinal cord. It is useful in the management of upper motor bladder dysfunction with external sphincter dyssynergia. Leyson et al. (1980) were able to demonstrate using urodynamic tests the ability of baclofen to decrease the external sphincter resistance in males with acute and chronic spinal cord injury. The residual urine was significantly reduced in 76% (19 of 25) of their cases within an average of 4.98 weeks. The usual adult dosage is 10 mg three times a day, which can be increased gradually to a maximum of 40–80 mg daily if necessary. The common

Table 5.4. Skeletal muscle relaxants

Drug	Preparation	Dosage[a]
Diazepam	5 and 10 mg tablets	5 mg t.i.d.–q.i.d. Paediatric: 0.2–0.4 mg/kg t.i.d.–q.i.d.
Baclofen	10 mg tablet	10 mg t.i.d.–q.i.d.
Dantrolene	25 mg tablet	25 mg t.i.d.

[a] Adult dosage unless otherwise specified. t.i.d., three times a day; q.i.d., four times a day.

side-effects include drowsiness, dizziness and muscle weakness. Abrupt termination of long-term therapy may be associated with visual and auditory hallucinations and agitated behaviour, and should be avoided.

Another group of skeletal muscle relaxants, represented by dantrolene (Dantrium), is those that affect the skeletal muscles directly. Dantrolene produces relaxation by interfering with the release of calcium ions from the sarcoplasmic reticulum. Pedersen et al. (1978) demonstrated the effect of intravenous dantrolene in four male patients with spastic paraplegia and hyperactive neurogenic bladder. Using a sphincterometric technique they observed a significant (29%) reduction in urethral resistance. Dantrolene has been suggested for use in detrusor sphincter dyssynergia, although experience is limited (Fig. 5.10). In a drug trial of oral dantrolene using an average dosage of 200–250 mg a day, Murdock et al. (1976) demonstrated excellent reduction of residual urine to less than 100 ml and improved radiographic appearance of the bladder outlet in all 6 cases treated for obstruction due to detrusor sphincter dyssynergia. The usual starting adult dosage is 25 mg three times a day. The dose can be increased as desired, but no more than 400 mg a day should be given. Dantrolene is contraindicated in patients with liver disease because it can induce fatal hepato-cellular injury in susceptible individuals. Common side-effects include drowsiness and dizziness. Long-term therapy may be associated with acne-like skin eruptions (Pinder et al. 1977).

Results with the use of skeletal muscle relaxants, as well as other agents including cholinergic drugs, have not been consistent. The failures observed with these medications may be due in part to the complexity of the different muscles and their innervation in the target organ. Gosling and co-workers (Gosling and Dixon 1979) have suggested that the skeletal muscle rhabdo-

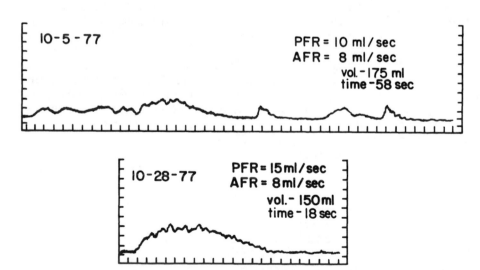

Fig. 5.10. Uroflow studies in a patient with detrusor sphincter dyssynergia secondary to multiple sclerosis. **a** The initial urine flow study demonstrates the interrupted weak stream. **b** A repeat uroflow study a month after dantrolene, substantiates the subjective improvement experienced by the patient.

sphincter of the urethra is innervated by the pelvic plexus rather than by the somatic pudendal nerve. This hypothesis would account for the inconsistent results encountered, while indicating a new approach to producing pharmacological relaxation of the sphincter.

Sympatholytic Agents: Internal Sphincter Relaxants (Table 5.5)

Phenoxybenzamine (Dibenzyline) is the drug usually used for relaxing the internal sphincter, and works by blocking alpha receptors in the smooth muscle of the vesical neck. It can be used either alone or in combination with cholinergic agents or even a skeletal muscle relaxant to improve emptying of the bladder. In combination therapy, a sympatholytic agent partially reduces urethral resistance, while a cholinergic agent increases detrusor pressure and a skeletal muscle relaxant further reduces the urethral resistance.

Table 5.5. Alpha-sympatholytic agents

Drug	Preparation	Dosage[a]
Phenoxybenzamine	10 mg capsule	10 mg t.i.d. Paediatric: 10 mg b.i.d.–t.i.d.
Prazosin	1 mg tablet	1 mg t.i.d.–q.i.d.

[a] Adult dosage unless otherwise specified. b.i.d., twice a day; t.i.d., three times a day; q.i.d., four times a day.

Krane and Olsson (1973) found phenoxybenzamine to be very successful in 6 patients with neurogenic detrusor/internal sphincter dyssynergia. In all reported cases the residual urine was reduced significantly. In 3 cases a combination of bethanechol and phenoxybenzamine was used to effect bladder emptying. Khanna and Gonick (1975) were able to demonstrate by studying the canine lower urinary tract, that this combination of drugs leads to an increase in the intravesical pressure and a lowering of the urethral and outlet pressure. In a series of 10 patients with functional outflow obstruction and atonic bladder evaluated urodynamically, Khanna (1976) obtained an excellent result in 8 patients by using 50–100 mg of bethanechol chloride with 20–30 mg of phenoxybenzamine daily.

The usual adult dosage of phenoxybenzamine is 10 mg three times a day and can be increased every 3 days to a maximum of 50–60 mg daily, or until side-effects become intolerable. The usual children's dosage is similar to the adult dosage, with a maximum of 10 mg three times a day. Children appear to tolerate the drug better than adults. The major side-effects are dizziness due to orthostatic hypotension, nasal congestion and retrograde ejaculation.

Prazosin (Minipress) is another alpha blocker that appears to be as effective as phenoxybenzamine and yet produces fewer side-effects. The alpha-adrenergic blocking properties of prazosin have been demonstrated in animal studies (MacGregor and Diokno 1981) and in the isolated human urethra (Andersson et al. 1981). In addition, in 7 patients with lower motor neuron lesions and micturition disturbances treated with prazosin, 5 had improved voiding, and the drug was shown to reduce the intra-urethral pressure. The starting dosage is 1 mg daily, which is gradually increased over 3–5 days to avoid the first-dose hypotension phenomenon seen with this drug. In our limited experience, we have used a maximum of 5 mg daily.

Alternative Treatments

Although drug therapy plays an important role as the sole treatment of neurogenic bladder dysfunction, it is important to emphasise that there are many instances where drug therapy is used as an adjunct to other therapeutic treatments.

In patients with uninhibited neurogenic bladders, the use of an anticholinergic agent is the primary form of treatment. However, it can also be used during bladder training programmes, to reduce the frequency of contractions and enlarge the bladder capacity. If pharmacological treatment and bladder training fail, surgical intervention such as bladder enlargement or denervation procedures can be considered.

In patients with reflex neurogenic bladders resulting from complete lesions above sacral segments 2–4, pharmacological therapy is generally used with other forms of therapy. For patients on intermittent catheterisation, anticholinergic agents are extremely useful for keeping the patient dry between catheterisations. In addition, for patients who have indwelling catheters, anticholinergic agents are helpful to prevent voiding around the catheter or extrusion of catheters with inflated balloons, and to avoid high intravesical pressures that can lead to vesico-ureteric reflux and sepsis. For those with reflex bladders who elect to wear a condom and empty their bladders spontaneously, the use of alpha blockers, skeletal muscle relaxants or cholinergic agents may be needed to effect complete emptying. For the dyssynergic, sphincterotomy should be considered if skeletal muscle relaxants are unsuccessful.

For patients with complete motor paralytic bladders, cholinergic therapy is completely ineffective. When the sphincters are preserved, intermittent catheterisation will be an ideal choice. When the sphincter is denervated, an alpha-adrenergic agent may be added to maintain continence. For those who fail in an intermittent catheterisation programme and have a paralysed sphincter, external catheter drainage or implantation of an artificial sphincter offer potential alternatives. Patients with preserved sphincter activity may require the addition of sphincterotomy to effect adequate bladder emptying. Patients with incompletely paralysed bladders are the only ones in this group who may benefit from a cholinergic agent.

In patients with a sensory paralytic bladder, frequent voiding by the clock may be all that is necessay. However, in the face of decompensation, intermittent catheterisation and/or cholinergic agents may be the treatment of choice.

In complex cases where both upper and lower motor lesions are present, combination therapy may be in order. For example, in the face of uncontrolled bladder contractions and a paralytic sphincter, as may be seen in lumbosacral lesions, both an anticholinergic and alpha-adrenergic agent may be necessary to maintain continence, while using intermittent catheterisation for bladder emptying. Alternatively, the use of an alpha blocker to improve emptying of the bladder with a Valsalva manoeuvre and the use of pads or condom catheters to collect the urine might better suit the patient's needs.

Autonomic Hyperreflexia (Table 5.6)

A discussion of the pharmacological therapy of the neuropathic bladder and sphincter would not be complete without mention of autonomic dysreflexia, often observed in quadriplegic and paraplegic patients with complete or incomplete lesions of thoracic segment 6 and higher. The syndrome usually results from bladder or rectal overdistension. The symptoms, which are mainly due to increased sympathetic discharge, are hypertension, headache, diaphoresis, flushing and bradycardia. Major complications such as cerebrovascular haemorrhage and even death have been reported.

Table 5.6. Drugs for autonomic hyperreflexia

Drug	Preparation	Dosage[a]
Sodium nitroprusside	50 mg/vial	50 mg/250 ml D5W; titrate dose (i.v.)
Trimetaphan	500 mg/ampule	500 mg/500 ml D5W; titrate dose (i.v.)
Guanethidine	10 mg tablet	10 mg t.i.d.
Phenoxybenzamine	10 mg capsule	10 mg t.i.d.

[a] D5W, 5% dextrose in water; i.v., intravenous; t.i.d., three times a day.

Emergency treatment involves immediate drainage of the distended viscus. If decompression is not accomplished immediately, or the blood pressure remains elevated, intravenous administration of a vascular smooth muscle relaxant such as nitroprusside (Nipride) or a ganglionic blocking agent such as trimetaphan camsylate (Arfonad) is effective. These drugs should always be on hand and ready to use when one is contemplating instrumentation or manipulation of the bladder of these patients. Sodium nitroprusside comes in 50 mg vials. It is mixed with 250 ml of 5% dextrose in water and the solution wrapped in an opaque wrapper such as aluminium foil to protect it from light. The average dose is 3 μg/kg per minute and should not exceed 10 μg/kg per minute. Trimetaphan camsylate comes in 500 mg vials, which are mixed with 500 ml of 5% dextrose in water. The average rate of infusion is 3–4 mg/minute. The exact dose should be titrated according to the blood pressure response. For chronic cases or as a prophylactic measure, guanethidine at a dosage of 10 mg three times a day can be used. Another alternative is phenoxybenzamine at a dosage of 10 mg orally three times a day. For chronic diaphoresis, oxybutynin (Ditropan) 5 mg orally three times a day is generally effective.

References

Andersson K-E, Ek A, Hedlund H, Mattiasson A (1981) Effects of prazosin on isolated human urethra and in patients with lower motor neuron lesions. Invest Urol 19:39–42

Awad SA, Bruce AW, Carro-Ciampi G, Downie JW, Lin M (1974) Distribution of alpha and beta adrenoceptors in human urinary bladder. Br J Pharmacol 50:525–529

Awad SA, Bryniak S, Downie JW, Bruce AW (1977) The treatment of the uninhibited bladder with dicyclomine. J Urol 117:161–163

Awad SA, Downie JW, Kiruluta HG (1978) Alpha-adrenergic agents in urinary disorders of the proximal urethra. II. Urethral obstruction due to 'sympathetic dyssynergia'. Br J Urol 50:336–339

Cannon WB, Rosenbleuth A (1949) The supersensitivity of denervated structures. Macmillan, New York

Diokno AC, Koppenhoefer R (1976) Bethanechol chloride in neurogenic bladder dysfunction. Urology 8:455–458

Diokno AC, Lapides J (1972) Oxybutynin, a new drug with analgesic and anticholinergic properties. J Urol 108:307–309

Diokno AC, Taub M (1975) Ephedrine in the treatment of urinary incontinence. Urology 5:624–625

Diokno AC, Koff SA, Bender LF (1974) Periurethral striated muscle activity in neurogenic bladder dysfunction. J Urol 112:743–749

Diokno AC, Davis R, Lapides J (1975) Urecholine test for denervated bladders. Invest Urol 13:233–235

Finkbeiner AE, Bissada NK (1980) Drug therapy for lower urinary tract dysfunction. Urol Clin North Am 7:3–16

Fischer CP, Diokno AC, Lapides J (1978) The anticholinergic effects of dicyclomine hydrochloride in uninhibited neurogenic bladder dysfunction. J Urol 120:328–329

Gosling JA, Dixon JS (1979) Light and electron microscopic observations on the human external urethral sphincter. J Anat 129:216

Gosling JA, Dixon JS, Critchley HOD, Thompson SA (1981) A comparative study of the human external sphincter and periurethral levator ani muscles. Br J Urol 53:35–41

Khanna OP (1976) Disorders of micturition: neuropharmacologic basis and results of drug therapy. Urology 8:316–328

Khanna OP, Gonick P (1975) Effects of phenoxybenzamine hydrochloride on canine lower urinary tract: clinical implication. Urology 6:323–330

Kieswetter H, Popper L (1972) A cystometrographic study to assess the influence of atropine, propantheline and mebeverine on the smooth muscle of the bladder. Br J Urol 44:31–35

Koff SA, Lapides, J, Piazza DH (1979) The uninhibited bladder in children: a cause for urinary obstruction, infection, and reflux. In: Hodson J, Kincaid-Smith P (eds) Reflux nephropathy. Masson Publishing, New York, pp 161–169

Koyanagi T, Tsuji I (1978) Reappraisal of the sympathetic role in the sphincteric urethra. Denervation supersensitivity of the urethra of the chronic neurogenic bladder to alpha-adrenergic drugs. Invest Urol 15:267–269

Krane RJ, Olsson CA (1973) Phenoxybenzamine in neurogenic bladder dysfunction. II. Clinical considerations. J Urol 110:653–656

Lapides J, Diokno AC (1976) Urine transport, storage and micturition. In: Lapides J (ed) Fundamental of urology. WB Saunders, Philadelphia, pp 190–241

Lapides J, Friend CR, Ajemian EP, Reus WS (1962) Denervation supersensitivity as a test for neurogenic bladder. Surg Gynecol Obstet 114:241–244

Leyson JFJ, Martin BF, Sporer A (1980) Baclofen in the Treatment of detrusor-sphincter dyssynergia in spinal cord injury patients. J Urol 124:82–84

MacGregor RJ, Diokno AC (1981) The alpha-adrenergic blocking action of prazosin hydrochloride on the canine urethra. Invest Urol 18:426–429

Murdock MM, Sax D, Krane RJ (1976) Use of dantrolene sodium in external sphincter spasm. Urology 8:133–137

Pedersen E, Harving H, Klemar B (1978) Effect of dantrolene sodium on the spastic external urethral sphincter recorded by sphincterometry. J Urol 119:403–405

Perlow DL, Diokno AC (1980) Cystometric and perineal electromyography in spinal cord-injured patients. Urology 15:432–433

Piazza DH, Diokno AC (1979) Review of neurogenic bladder in multiple sclerosis. Urology 14:33–35

Pinder RM, Brogden RN, Speight TM, Avery GS (1977) Dantrolene sodium: a review of its pharmacological properties and therapeutic efficacy in spasticity. Drugs 13:3–23

Raz S, Bradley WE (1979) Neuromuscular dysfunction of the lower urinary tract. In: Harrison JH et al. (eds) Urology, 4th edn. WB Saunders, Philadelphia, pp 1215–1270

Smey P, Firlit CF, King LR (1978) Voiding pattern abnormalities in normal children: results of pharmacologic manipulation. J Urol 120:574–577

Sonda LP, Gershon C, Diokno AC, Lapides J (1979) Further observations on the cystometric and uroflowmetric effects of bethanechol chloride on the human bladder. J Urol 122:775–777

Sporer A, Leyson JFJ, Martin BF (1978) Effects of bethanechol chloride on the external urethral sphincter in spinal cord injury patients. J Urol 120:62–66

Stewart BH, Banowsky LHW, Montague DK (1976) Stress incontinence: conservative therapy with sympathomimetic drugs. J Urol 115:558–559

Thompson IM, Lauvetz R (1976) Oxybutynin in bladder spasm, neurogenic bladder and enuresis. Urology 8:452–454

Vaidyanathan A, Rao MS, Mapa MK, Bapna BC, Chary KSN, Swamy RP (1981) Study of intravesical instillation of 15-(S)-15 methyl prostaglandin $F_{2\alpha}$ in patients with neurogenic bladder dysfunction. J Urol 126:81–85

Vinson RK, Diokno AC (1976) Uninhibited neurogenic bladder in adults. Urology 7:376–378

Yalla SV, Rossier AB, Fam B (1976) Dyssynergic vesicourethral responses during bladder rehabilitation in spinal cord injury patients: effects of suprapubic percussion, Credé method and bethanechol chloride. J Urol 115:575–579

Chapter 6

Pharmacological Treatment of Non-neurogenic Voiding Dysfunction

Alan J. Wein

Introduction

The lower urinary tract performs two functions: the storage and emptying of urine. The physiology of the cycle of micturition has been described by many qualified authors, each of whom has given his own particular concept of the neuroanatomy and neurophysiology of the smooth and striated muscular structures, the peripheral autonomic and somatic neural factors, and the spinal and supraspinal influences which are necessary for the normal micturition cycle. There are significant disagreements regarding the finer details of the relevant neuromorphology, neurophysiology and neuropharmacology. Perhaps the best example of this is the current controversy over the influence of the sympathetic nervous system on the physiology of micturition and the interrelationships, if any, of the parasympathetic and sympathetic influences on the smooth muscle of the urinary bladder and its outlet.

It is important to realise that exact agreement regarding the neuromorphological and neurophysiological details is *not* necessary for an understanding of the pharmacological principles involved in drug-induced alteration of voiding function. Although there are these differences in the interpretation of data concerning lower urinary tract function, all of these authors would doubtless agree that voiding function, and therefore voiding dysfunction, can be described in terms of a relatively discrete filling–storage phase and an emptying phase (Wein and Raezer 1979). Urinary continence and the normal storage of urine during bladder filling require: (1) accommodation of increasing volumes of urine at a low intravesical pressure and with appropriate sensory appreciation; (2) a bladder outlet which is closed at rest and remains so during increases in intra-abdominal pressure; and (3) the absence of involuntary bladder contractions (bladder instability or detrusor hyperreflexia). Normal urine emptying requires (1) a coordinated bladder contraction of sufficient magnitude; (2) absence of anatomical obstruction; and (3) a concomitant lowering of resistance at the level of the smooth muscle of the bladder neck and proximal urethra (the so-called smooth sphincter) and at the level of the striated musculature comprising the external urethral sphincter (the so-called striated sphincter). All types of therapy for voiding dysfunction, neurogenic or non-neurogenic, can be classified within a functional scheme which is derived from these simple concepts (Tables 6.1 and 6.2). This chapter will discuss in general the evaluation of pharmacological agents in the treatment of voiding dysfunction and will summarise, using this classification, current thought regarding the efficacy of various types of pharmacotherapy for disorders of micturition.

The pharmacological principles and explanations are the same whether one is dealing with voiding dysfunction secondary to a neurological lesion or not. Thus, overlap is inevitable between this chapter and Chap. 5 which describes pharmacotherapy for neurogenic voiding dysfunction. Pharmacotherapy for bladder outlet obstruction secondary to benign prostatic hypertrophy is covered exclusively in Chapter 7.

Table 6.1. Therapy to facilitate bladder emptying

A. Increase intravesical pressure
   1. External compression
   2. Promotion or initiation of reflex contractions
      (a) Trigger zones or manoeuvres
      (b) Bladder training, tidal drainage
   3. Pharmacological manipulation
      (a) Parasympathomimetic agents
      (b) Blockers of inhibition (?)
      (c) Prostaglandins
   4. Electrical stimulation
      (a) Directly to the bladder
      (b) To the nerve root or spinal cord

B. Decrease outlet resistance
   1. At the level of the bladder neck
      (a) Transurethral resection or incision
      (b) Y-V 'plasty
      (c) Pharmacological inhibition (alpha-adrenergic blockade)
   2. At the level of the distal mechanism[a]
      (a) External sphincterotomy
      (b) Urethral overdilation
      (c) Pudendal nerve interruption
      (d) Pharmacological inhibition
         I. External sphincter/pelvic floor (striated muscle relaxant)
         II. Proximal urethra (alpha-adrenergic blockade)
      (e) Psychotherapy, biofeedback

C. Circumvent problem
   1. Intermittent catheterisation
   2. Urinary diversion

[a] Distal mechanism refers to the smooth muscle of the proximal urethra together with the external (striated muscle) urethral sphincter. This terminology is that of Turner-Warwick, who divides the components of the continence mechanism in male and female into proximal (bladder neck) and distal elements.

Table 6.2. Therapy to facilitate urine storage

A. Inhibit bladder contractility
    1. Pharmacological manipulation
        (a) Anticholinergic agents
        (b) Beta-adrenergic stimulation
        (c) Musculotropic relaxants
        (d) Polysynaptic inhibitors
        (e) Calcium antagonists
        (f) Prostaglandin inhibitors
    2. Interruption of innervation
        (a) Subarachnoid block
        (b) Sacral rhizotomy
        (c) Bladder denervation (peripheral)
    3. Bladder overdistension
    4. Cystolysis
    5. Electrical stimulation (reflex inhibition)
    6. Cystoplasty[a]

B. Increase outlet resistance
    1. At the level of the bladder neck
        (a) Alpha-adrenergic stimulation
        (b) Mechanical compression
    2. At the level of the distal mechanism
        (a) Alpha-adrenergic stimulation, beta-adrenergic blockade (?)
        (b) Mechanical compression
        (c) Electrical stimulation of the pelvic floor

C. Circumvent problem
    1. Intermittent catheterisation
    2. Urinary diversion

---

[a] This procedure primarily augments bladder capacity and only secondarily inhibits bladder contractility by raising the volume thresholds for sensation and distension.

Principles of Pharmacotherapy for Voiding Dysfunction: Evaluation of Drug Effects on Lower Urinary Tract Function

To use any pharmacological agent intelligently, it is necessary to be familiar not only with its biochemical and physiological effects and mechanisms of action, but also with all those factors which determine its concentration at its site of action. Additionally, one must be thoroughly familiar with the literature surrounding the use of a particular agent and remember that:

1) An agent may act at more than one site and even at several sites within a neural pathway or muscle, and each of these effects may have a different net action on the function generally performed by the final effector.

2) An agent may have different effects in vitro and in vivo, and in the same system at different concentrations.

3) An agent may have different effects in different species.

4) An agent may have different acute and long-term effects.

5) If an agent has multiple effects at different levels of action, each may occur at a different time.

6) The sensitivity, number and type of receptors within a particular tissue can be affected by its physiological state (denervation, distension, hypertrophy, inflammation, ischaemia) and by the pharmacological agent itself.

Generally speaking, the simplest and least hazardous pharmacological agent within a given category should be tried first. If single-agent therapy fails, a combination of therapeutic manoeuvres or pharmacological agents can sometimes be used to achieve a particular effect, especially if the mechanisms of action are different and the side-effects are not synergistic.

Although a number of clinical trials in the literature are of high quality, many have deficiencies in design, conduct, analysis, or presentation of results. This is especially true for non-neurogenic voiding dysfunction, where the urodynamic correlates seem to be less constant from day to day than in patients with a fixed neurological lesion. Most investigators would agree that an ideal clinical trial of a pharmacological agent for treatment of a particular condition should satisfy certain general criteria (Fingl and Woodbury 1975; Wein 1981):

1) Lack of bias
2) Inclusion of an adequate number of subjects
3) Use of appropriate and sensitive methods of evaluation
4) Double-blind conditions with a placebo
5) Statistical validation.

Appropriate and sensitive methodology should include objective as well as subjective criteria. Ideally, these methods will yield objective urodynamic data which are easily subject to statistical analysis. Subjective data, usually in the form of symptoms, are generally difficult to quantify and analyse. A prospective randomised double-blind study is the ideal method for determining the clinical efficacy of a therapeutic intervention. Such a design virtually eliminates bias, and, with an adequate sample size, ensures, as far as possible, that the results obtained are due to factors other than sampling variability. Regarding protocols which use primarily subjective criteria for assessment, it has long been recognised that improvement in such criteria may occur in up to 35% of placebo-treated patients (Benson and Epstein 1975). In general, such a placebo effect can be boosted by a very positive and enthusiastic attitude on the part of the treating physician, by the length of time spent with the patient, and by an in-hospital type of regimen. If a drug is clinically effective it should be compared, over pharmacological dose ranges, with a 'reference' drug in terms of effectiveness, selectivity, side-effects and cost.

Failure to Empty

Pathophysiology, Symptomatology and General Outline of Treatment

Absolute or relative failure to empty results from decreased bladder contractility, increased outlet resistance, or both. Absolute or relative failure of adequate bladder contractility may result from temporary or permanent alteration in any one of the neuromuscular mechanisms necessary for initiating and maintaining a normal detrusor contraction. Non-neurogenic causes include impairment of the bladder smooth muscle which may result from overdistension, severe infection or fibrosis. Inhibition of the micturition reflex in a neurologically normal individual may occur via a reflex mechanism secondary to painful stimuli, especially from the pelvic and perineal areas. Increased outlet resistance is generally secondary to anatomical obstruction, or to a failure of adequate relaxation of the striated sphincter or of proper adaptive changes in the area of the smooth sphincter.

Urinary retention is the obvious symptomatic end-point of a total failure to empty. Hesitancy and straining to void generally reflect relative failure. Inadequate bladder emptying may also be associated with overflow urinary incontinence. Increased urinary frequency may likewise result from a failure to empty, due to a decreased functional bladder capacity caused by a substantial residual urine volume. Although symptoms can be strongly suggestive of the primary type of voiding dysfunction present, they are often misleading, and therefore a thorough urodynamic evaluation is generally encouraged before the institution of treatment. Treatment for failure to empty generally consists of attempts to increase intravesical pressure, decrease outlet resistance, or both.

Pharmacotherapy to Increase Intravesical Pressure

Parasympathomimetic Agents

Although it is likely that other excitatory neurotransmitters exist, it is agreed that at least a major portion of the final common pathway in physiological bladder contraction is acetylcholine-induced stimulation of the muscarinic–cholinergic receptor sites at the postganglionic parasympathetic neuromuscular junction (Wein and Raezer 1979). Thus, agents which imitate the actions of acetylocholine might be expected to be useful in the management of any patient who exhibits a failure to empty because of inadequate bladder contractility. Acetylcholine itself cannot be used for therapeutic purposes because of actions at the central and ganglionic levels, as well as at the peripheral neuromuscular junction, and because of its rapid hydrolysis by acetylcholinesterase and by non-specific cholinesterase (Koelle 1975).

There are many agents which imitate the action of acetylcholine on smooth muscle. However, only bethanechol chloride is reported to exhibit a relatively selective action on the urinary bladder and gut with little or no action at therapeutic doses on ganglia or on the cardiovascular system (Ursillo 1967; Koelle 1975). Bethanechol chloride is cholinesterase-resistant and in vitro causes contraction of smooth muscle from bladder body and base (Raezer et al. 1973). Its use in the treatment of post-operative urinary retention was first reported by Starr and Ferguson (1940) and current recommendations in this regard are for subcutaneous doses of 5–10 mg in an awake, alert patient with no outlet obstruction. It has been used in the treatment of the atonic or hypotonic bladder for over 30 years (Lee 1949) and has been reported as effective in achieving 'rehabilitation' of the chronically atonic or hypotonic detrusor (Lapides 1964, 1974; Diokno and Koppenhoefer 1976; Sonda et al. 1979). For this purpose, it is recommended that the drug be initially administered subcutaneously at a dosage of 5–10 mg (usually 7.5 mg) every 4–6 hours. This is initiated with the patient preferably on intermittent catheterisation. The patient is asked to try and void 20–30 minutes after each subcutaneous dose and, when the residual urine has decreased to an acceptable level, the dose is decreased by 2.5 mg and ultimately changed to an oral dosage of 50 mg four times daily. In cases of partial bladder emptying, a therapeutic trial of an oral dosage of 25–100 mg four times daily is used in conjunction with attempted voiding every 4 hours with abdominal straining and credé.

Although bethanechol has been accepted by some as an agent which increases gastro-intestinal motility (Kilbinger and Weihrauch 1982) and which is useful for the treatment of gastro-oesophageal reflux (Richter and Castell 1982), attempts to facilitate bladder emptying in patients where bethanechol was the only variable have been urodynamically disappointing. Using a pharmacologically active subcutaneous dose (5 mg) we were unable to demonstrate significant changes in flow parameters or residual urine either in 12 women with a residual urine volume equal to or greater than 20% of bladder capacity but no evidence of neurological disease or outlet obstruction, or 27 'normal' women of approximately the same mean age (Wein et al. 1980b). A similar dose also failed to produce urodynamic evidence of improved emptying in patients with a positive bethanechol supersensitivity test (Wein et al. 1980a). This dosage did increase the intravesical pressure at all points along the filling limb of the cystometrogram, and also decreased the bladder capacity threshold, findings previously described by others (Lapides et al. 1963; Sonda et al. 1979). Although bethanechol chloride in adequate doses is capable of eliciting an increase in tension in bladder smooth muscle, such as one would expect from in vitro studies, we remain unimpressed with its ability to stimulate or facilitate a true physiological type of bladder contraction in the vast majority of patients with neurogenic or non-neurogenic disease.

Similar sentiments, at least with respect to its use in neurogenic bladder dysfunction, have been expressed by Gibbon (1965), Merrill and Rotta (1974) and Yalla et al. (1977). It is difficult to find reproducible urodynamic data which support the use of bethanechol chloride in any category of patients who exhibit a failure to empty. Invariably, long-term studies in such patients are neither prospective nor double-blind and do not exclude the effects of other simultaneous regimens, such as treatment of urinary infection, bladder decompression by continuous or intermittent catheterisation, or timed voiding with credé. Short-term studies in which the drug was the only variable have generally failed to demonstrate significant benefit in terms of flow and residual urine volume data.

It is generally agreed, even by proponents of the use of bethanechol, that oral doses of 50 mg or less have little, if any, effect on even cystometric parameters (Diokno and Lapides 1977; Wein et al. 1978). More recently, Barrett (1981) has shown no significant difference in urodynamic parameters in patients given a single dose of 0, 25, 50 or 100 mg of oral medication. These were female patients with residual urine volumes greater than 125 ml without evidence of neurological disease or bladder outlet obstruction. He likewise failed to show any improvement in flowmetry or residual urine volume. It is generally agreed that, at least in a denervated bladder, an oral dose of 200 mg is required to produce the same effect as a subcutaneous dose of 5 mg (Diokno and Lapides 1977; Philp et al. 1980). Whether repeated doses of bethanechol or any other cholinergic agonist can achieve a clinical effect that a single dose cannot is speculative. If such is not the case, the long-term response to therapy could be predicted by a urodynamic assessment before and after a single subcutaneous dose or a short oral trial.

Other methods of achieving a cholinergic effect are seldom used in the United States. Philp et al. (1980) reported that a 4 mg oral dose of carbachol, a cholinergic agonist which possesses also some ganglionic stimulating properties, had a much greater effect on urodynamic parameters than a 50 mg oral dose of bethanechol, without an apparent increase in side-effects. Anticholinesterase agents, which inhibit the enzymatic degradation of acetylcholine, also have the net effect of producing or enhancing cholinergic stimulation. Cameron (1966) found that distigmine bromide, a long-acting anticholinesterase, was effective in preventing post-operative urinary retention. Philp and Thomas (1980) have reported that parenteral, but not oral, distigmine improved voiding efficiency in patients with neurogenic bladder dysfunction with reflex detrusor activity. They recommended an intramuscular dosage of 0.5 mg a day. It is also available as a 5 mg oral preparation.

In those patients in whom cholinergic stimulation does seem to improve voiding efficiency, one may speculate that it does so by causing reflex contraction or the sensation of distension at a lower bladder volume than usual, thereby allowing a contraction to occur at a muscle fibre length more favourable to the development of a strong coordinated contraction.

There is no agreement as to whether cholinergic stimulation produces an increase in urethral resistance (Wein 1980; Wein et al. 1980b). It would appear that pharmacologically active doses do in fact increase urethral closure pressure, at least in patients with neurogenic bladder dysfunction with detrusor hyperreflexia (Sporer et al. 1978). If such a phenomenon does occur, a logical question would be whether emptying could be facilitated by combining cholinergic agonists with agents that decrease outlet resistance. Khanna (1976) reported that a combination of a total daily oral dose of bethanechol of 50–100 mg with 20–30 mg of oral phenoxybenzamine (see section on decreasing outlet resistance, p. 108ff.) produced what he termed satisfactory results in a group of patients with an atonic bladder and functional outlet obstruction. Our own experience in this situation with even combined pharmacological therapy such as this has been extremely disappointing. Certainly, most would agree that this particular oral dose of bethanechol rarely affects any urodynamic measurement (Lapides et al. 1963; Diokno and Lapides 1977; Wein et al. 1978; Philp et al. 1980).

The potential side-effects of the cholinergic agonists and the anticholinesterase agents are similar and include flushing, nausea, vomiting, diarrhoea, gastro-intestinal cramps, bronchospasm, headache, salivation, sweating, and difficulty with visual accommodation. Intramuscular or intravenous use of bethanechol is contraindicated, as it can precipitate acute and severe side-effects resulting in acute circulatory failure and cardiac arrest. Contraindications for the use of these general categories of drug include bronchial asthma, peptic ulcer, bowel obstruction, enteritis, history of recent gastro-intestinal surgery, cardiac arrhythmia, hyperthyroidism, or any type of bladder outlet obstruction (Koelle 1975; Wein 1979).

Prostaglandins

The role of prostaglandins in lower urinary tract physiology is undergoing active investigation. Bultitude et al. (1976) hypothesised that prostaglandins and acetylcholine were both necessary for the maintenance of bladder tone and spontaneous bladder activity. They summarised their supporting evidence as follows: (1) prostaglandins were produced by the bladder; (2) the prostaglandins PGE_2 and $PGF_{2\alpha}$ caused a dose-related contraction in bladder strips in vitro; and (3) inhibitors of prostaglandin synthesis caused a decrease in bladder tone and spontaneous activity. This group reported that instillation of 0.5 mg PGE_2 into the bladders of females with varying degrees of urinary retention resulted in acute emptying and improved long-term emptying in two-thirds of the patients studied.

Desmond et al. (1980) reported further results with this agent in patients whose bladders exhibited no contractile activity or in whom bladder contractility was relatively impaired. A dose of 1.5 mg of PGE_2 in diluent was infused intravesically and left for 1 hour. Twenty of 36 patients showed a strongly positive, and 6 a weakly positive immediate response. Fourteen patients, all but one of whom had shown a strongly positive immediate response, showed prolonged beneficial effects. Stratification of the data revealed that an intact sacral reflex arc was a prerequisite for any type of positive response. The authors noted additionally that the effects of PGE_2 appeared to be additive or synergistic with cholinergic stimulation in some patients.

In contrast, other investigators, including Stanton (1978) and Delaere et al. (1981), have reported no success with this type of treatment. The latter group used doses of PGE_2 ranging from 0.5 to 10 mg and doses of $PGF_{2\alpha}$ ranging from 1 to 5 mg. Prostaglandins have a relatively short half-life and it is difficult to understand how any effects after a single application can last up to even several months. If such an action does occur, it must be the result of a 'triggering effect' on some as yet undescribed physiological metabolic mechanism. PGE_2 is not available in the United States in anything other than a rectal suppository form. $PGF_{2\alpha}$ is available in an injectable form, but guidelines for its use do not at present include voiding dysfunction. Potential side-effects of prostaglandin usage include bronchospasm, chills, hypotension, tachycardia, cardiac arrhythmia, convulsions, hypocalcaemia and diarrhoea (Moncada et al. 1980).

Blockers of Inhibition

de Groat and coworkers (de Groat and Saum 1972, 1976; de Groat and Booth 1980) have demonstrated a sympathetic reflex which, at least in the cat, promotes urine storage by exerting an inhibitory effect on pelvic parasympathetic ganglionic transmission. This effect, although inhibitory, is alpha-adrenergic in nature. Some have suggested on this basis that alpha-adrenergic blockade may, in addition to decreasing outlet resistance (see next section), facilitate transmission through these ganglia and thereby enhance bladder contractility. Guanethidine (Hartviksen 1966) and methyldopa (Raz et al. 1977) have been used with this rationale with at least some good results, but subsequent reports supporting these findings have not appeared. Raz and Smith (1976), using this same rationale, have advocated a trial of phenoxybenzamine for the treatment of non-obstructive urinary retention. Some clinicians, ourselves included, have anecdotally reported success using this or some other exotic approach, but we would caution against the assumption, without a controlled clinical study, that improvement in such a situation while *on* a drug occurs solely *because of* it.

Pharmacotherapy to Decrease Outlet Resistance

At the Level of the Smooth Sphincter

The observation that sympatholytic drugs are capable of facilitating emptying in certain patients was first made by Kleeman in 1970. Krane and Olsson (1973a,b) described the concept of a physiological internal sphincter, controlled partially by tonic stimulation of these contractile alpha receptors in the smooth musculature of the bladder neck and proximal urethra via the sympathetic nervous system. Further, they hypothesised that some obstructions which occur at this level during detrusor contraction are a result of inadequate opening of the bladder neck or/and an inadequate decrease in resistance in the area of the proximal urethra. They also theorised and presented evidence that alpha-adrenergic blockade could be useful in promoting emptying in such a patient with an adequate bladder contraction but without anatomical obstruction or detrusor–striated sphincter dyssynergia. They selected six such cases for presentation, five of which showed satisfactory voiding patterns 1 to 15 months after therapy with the alpha-adrenergic blocking agent phenoxybenzamine, the therapy having been initiated during a short period of catheter drainage. In the sixth patient, treatment was discontinued because of orthostatic hypotension.

Abel et al. (1974) called attention to the fact that such a functional obstruction, which they too presumed to be activated by the sympathetic nervous system, could be maximal in the urethra, rather than at the bladder neck, coining the term 'the neuropathic urethra'. The implication that alpha-adrenergic blockade could be useful in certain patients with a failure to empty despite an adequate increase in intravesical pressure was subsequently supported by others (Johnston and Farkas 1975; Stockamp 1975; Stockamp and Schreiter 1975; Whitfield et al. 1976). Successful results, usually defined as an increase in flow rate, decrease in residual urine, and improved upper tract appearance (where pathological) could often be correlated with an objective decrease in urethral profile closure pressures.

In addition to the effect on smooth muscle, it has been suggested that alpha-adrenergic blocking agents may decrease perineal striated muscle activity and that this action may contribute to their effect in decreasing outlet resistance (Nanninga et al. 1977). If this is so, it would seem that such a mechanism must be a central one, or must be mediated by non-innervated receptors, as adrenergic innervation of the striated urethral sphincter appears to be lacking (Wein et al. 1979; Rossier et al. 1982).

The phentolamine stimulation test (Olsson et al. 1977) can usually predict the effectiveness of alpha-adrenolytic therapy in a given situation. Flow rates are measured before and after an intravenous dose of 5 mg, and the values are plotted on a nomogram which relates flow rate to volume voided. An increase of 0.8 units on the nomogram predicts improved voiding with oral alpha blockers.

There has been a group of patients, predominantly male, without neurological disease or anatomical obstruction of any type who exhibit a failure to empty despite an adequate bladder contraction and a lack of striated sphincter dyssynergia. These patients, adult and paediatric, can often have their condition improved with alpha-adrenergic blocking agents, and their voiding dysfunction has variously been termed bladder neck dysfunction, bladder neck dyssynergy, internal sphincter dyssynergia, and smooth sphincter dyssynergy (Turner-Warwick et al. 1973; Smey et al. 1980; Kaneko et al. 1980).

Phenoxybenzamine is the alpha-adrenolytic agent most commonly used in the treatment of voiding dysfunction (Wein 1979, 1980). The initial adult dosage of this agent is 10 mg daily. An electrocardiogram and supine and standing blood pressure measurements are recommended before initiating therapy. The dose may be increased by 10 mg every 4–5 days to a recommended maximum of 60 mg daily. Daily doses larger than 10 mg are generally divided and given every 8–12 hours. The maximum effect of a particular dose usually becomes apparent only after a week of therapy. After discontinuing the therapy, the effects of daily administration persist for about the same period of time. In our experience, patients who respond favourably to this agent generally do so at doses less than 30 mg and do not respond to dose increases with incremental improvement. Some patients who respond to 10 mg daily can be maintained on an even lower dose. Potential side-effects include orthostatic hypotension, reflex tachycardia, nasal congestion, diarrhoea, miosis, sedation, nausea and vomiting (secondary to local irritation) (Weiner 1980b). Ejaculatory failure, due to lack of seminal emission and not to retrograde ejaculation, frequently occurs (Kedia and Persky 1981), but without any adverse effect on erection.

Those who use phenoxybenzamine should be aware of the recently reported adverse in vitro and in vivo mutagenicity studies (McNally 1982). These reports indicate that it produced increases in gene mutation in in vitro systems employing salmonella bacteria and mouse lymphoma cells, but that it did not increase the frequency of micronuclei in mouse bone marrow cells in vivo. The manufacturer has started a 2-year carcinogenicity study in rats to provide a more definite answer as to the carcinogenic potential of phenoxybenzamine. Although this agent has been in use for some 30 years in humans without any startling epidemiological associations, it is obvious that the results of the current long-term carcinogenicity studies are anxiously awaited.

Prazosin hydrochloride is one of a new class of antihypertensive agents with an affinity for post-synaptic alpha-1 receptors, at least in vascular smooth muscle (Atkins and Nicolosi 1979; Graham and Pettinger 1979; Weiner 1980c). This agent has little affinity for alpha-2 receptors, in contrast to the classical alpha-adrenergic blocking agents such as phentolamine and phenoxybenzamine, both of which have blocking properties at alpha-1 and alpha-2 receptor sites. Prazosin has been shown to cause alpha-1 blockade in the smooth muscle of the canine and human urethra (MacGregor and Diokno 1981; Andersson et al. 1981). In this respect, it is theoretically preferable to phenoxybenzamine because of its relatively selective postsynaptic action. At least with respect to equivalent hypotensive doses, phenoxybenzamine produces a greater increase in plasma noradrenaline concentration than prazosin. Consistent with this, the reported incidence of reflex tachycardia with phenoxybenzamine is greater.

Therapy with prazosin is generally begun in daily divided doses of 2–3 mg. The dose may be very gradually increased to a maximum of 20 mg daily.

The dose of this agent which is equivalent to the 'standard' 10 mg dose of phenoxybenzamine for voiding dysfunction is as yet unknown. The potential side-effects of prazosin are consequent to its alpha-1 blockade. Additionally, there occasionally occurs the 'first-dose phenomenon', a symptom complex of faintness, dizziness, palpitation and, occasionally, syncopy. These episodes, when they occur, generally happen within 30–90 minutes of the first dose, and are thought to be due to acute postural hypotension. The incidence of this phenomenon can be minimised by restricting the initial dose of the drug to 1 mg and by administering this at bedtime. Other side-effects associated with chronic prazosin therapy are generally mild and rarely necessitate withdrawal of the drug (Graham and Pettinger 1979). Thus far, reports of adverse effects on seminal emission have been sparse.

Other agents with some alpha-adrenergic blocking properties at various levels of neural organisation have urological side-effects which may be therapeutically useful in certain circumstances. Methyldopa is an antihypertensive agent which is converted to alphamethylnoradrenaline; this functions as a false neuro-transmitter at a central and perhaps peripheral level, the end result being a decreased peripheral sympathetic effect (Weinshilboum 1980; Blaschke and Melmon 1980). Raz et al. (1977) have reported improved emptying in patients with neurogenic bladder dysfunction with this agent. Clonidine is another anti-hypertensive agent whose net effect is a decreased peripheral sympathetic effect, reflected in the urinary tract by a decrease in the urethral closure pressure profile (Nordling et al. 1979). This agent appears to produce an initial direct stimulation of peripheral alpha-1 receptors followed by a significant decrease in sympathetic neural traffic from the central nervous system, a phenomenon which may or may not be related to its action as an alpha-adrenergic agonist with relative specificity for alpha-2 receptor sites (Krier et al. 1979; Weinshilboum 1980; Weiner 1980c; Blaschke and Melmon 1980). Other commonly used pharmacological agents with significant alpha-adrenergic blocking properties include chlorpromazine and haloperidol (Weiner 1980c). Ron et al. (1980) have also reported an alpha-1 blocking property of bromocriptine in the lower urinary tract, although this agent has been reported to be an alpha-2 agonist in low doses in an isolated artery preparation (Ziegler et al. 1979).

Beta-adrenergic stimulation has been shown experimentally to decrease the urethral pressure profile and by inference urethral resistance (Raz and Caine 1972). The beta receptors of urethral smooth muscle are of the beta-2 type, producing a decrease in smooth muscle tension upon stimulation. This accounts for the decrease in urethral closure pressure after administration of terbutaline, a relatively specific beta-2 agonist (Vaidyanathan et al. 1980). Whether this drug or other pharmacologically similar agents will prove useful in facilitating bladder emptying by decreasing outlet resistance remains to be investigated.

At the Level of the Striated Sphincter

Classical detrusor striated sphincter dyssynergia is generally seen only in patients with overt neurological damage between the brainstem and sacral spinal cord. A disorder that is at least qualitatively similar can be seen in patients without an apparent structural or neurological basis and falls into what Hinman (1980) described as one of the syndromes of incoordination (Hinman 1974; Raz and Smith 1976; Allen 1977).

There is no class of pharmacological agents which will selectively relax the striated musculature of the pelvic floor. Chlordiazepoxide, methocarbamol, orphenadrine, and diazepam belong to a group of agents classified as centrally acting muscle relaxants (Franz 1975). Effective total daily doses of diazepam, the most widely used agent of this group, range from 6 to 60 mg. The primary side-effect of all members of this group is sedation, which many feel is primarily responsible for their muscle-relaxing effect when administered orally. Only a few studies have actually shown any advantage of these agents, as regards their relaxing effect purely on striated muscle over a placebo or aspirin (Byck 1975). In fact, oral diazepam is classified primarily as an anti-anxiety therapy by some authorities (Byck 1975). In general, we have not found the recommended oral doses to be effective in controlling the classical type of striated sphincter dyssynergia secondary to true neurological disease. If the aetiology of incomplete emptying in a neurologically normal patient is obscure, and the patient has what appears to be inadequate relaxation of the pelvic floor striated musculature, a trial of an agent such as diazepam may be worthwhile. The rationale is either that of relaxation of the pelvic floor striated musculature during bladder contraction, or such relaxation removing an inhibitory stimulus to bladder activity. Improvement under such circumstances may simply be due, however, to the drug's anti-anxiety effect or to the intensive explanation, encouragement, and modified biofeedback therapy which usually accompanies this type of treatment in such patients.

Dantrolene sodium is a skeletal muscle relaxant which has been shown to dissociate excitation–contraction coupling at a site distal to the neuromuscular end-plate in the sarcoplasmic reticulm (Franz 1975). It has been shown to have therapeutic benefits in chronic spasticity associated with central nervous system disorders. The drug has been used in patients with classical detrusor–striated sphincter dyssynergia, and was initially reported as being rather successful in improving voiding function in these patients (Murdock et al. 1976). It is recommended that adult therapy begins at a dosage of 25 mg twice daily, increasing weekly by 50–100 mg increments up to a daily maximum of 400 mg given in divided doses. Hackler et al. (1980) achieved improvement in voiding function in approximately half of their patients treated with dantrolene, but found that improvement required doses of 600 mg per day. Although the drug has no autonomic side-effects, it may induce a generalised weakness severe enough to compromise its therapeutic benefits, especially at higher doses. Other potential side-effects include euphoria, dizziness, diarrhoea and hepatotoxicity, the latter apparently being related to long-term usage of high doses. Because of the variable therapeutic success of this agent, some have speculated that it might adversely affect bladder smooth muscle contractility. However, Harris and Benson (1980) have shown quite conclusively that no such inhibitory action on bladder smooth muscle occurs.

Baclofen is an agent which is a derivative of gamma-aminobutyric acid, an inhibitory spinal cord neurotransmitter, and causes inhibition of mono- and polysynaptic spinal reflex activity (Jones et al. 1970; Duncan et al. 1976). Additionally, it may cause a depression of the synaptic relay of the primary afferent fibres in the dorsal column nuclei (Fox et al. 1978). It has been found useful in the treatment of skeletal spasticity due to a variety of causes (Roussan et al. 1975; Abromowicz 1978). Treatment is started at an initial dosage of 5 mg three times daily, and the dose is doubled every 3 days until a daily total dose level of 60 mg is reached. The manufacturer recommends that the total daily dose does not exceed 20 mg four times daily. Hachen and Krucker (1977) found a 75 mg daily oral dose to be ineffective in patients with striated sphincter dyssynergia and traumatic paraplegia, whereas a daily intravenous dose of 20 mg was highly effective. Leyson et al. (1980) reported that 73% of their patients with voiding dysfunction secondary to acute and chronic spinal cord injury showed lowered striated sphincter responses and decreased residual urine volume following treatment with an average daily oral dose of 120 mg. Potential side-effects of baclofen include drowsiness, insomnia, rash, pruritis, dizziness and weakness. Hallucinations may sometimes occur after abrupt withdrawal.

Beta-adrenergic agonists, especially those with predominant beta-2 character-istics, are also able to produce relaxation of some skeletal muscles of the slow twitch type (Olsson et al. 1979; Holmberg and Waldeck 1980). This may be especially significant in view of the fact that Gosling et al. (1981) have reported that portion of the external urethral sphincter which comprises the outermost urethral wall to consist exclusively of slow twitch fibres, while the striated muscle fibres of the levator ani contain both fast twitch and slow twitch fibres, although the majority are of the slow twitch type. This type of action may account at least in part for the decrease in urethral profile parameters seen with terbutaline, a relatively specific beta-2 agonist, and may form the basis for further attempts with such agents to decrease outlet resistance (Vaidyanathan et al. 1980).

Failure to Store

Pathophysiology, Symptomatology and General Outline of Treatment

The pathophysiology of failure to store urine adequately may be secondary to reasons related to the bladder, the outlet, or both. Hyperactivity of the bladder during filling can be expressed as involuntary contractions or decreased compli-ance. Involuntary contractions may occur with the sensation of impending micturition or urgency, but may occur without sensory awareness. Involuntary contractions are most commonly seen in association with neurological disease or injury, but may also be associated with bladder outlet obstruction, inflamma-tory or irritative processes in the bladder itself, or may be idiopathic.

The exact aetiology of the hyperreflexia which develops in response to bladder outlet obstruction is as yet unknown. This phenomenon has been best described in association with anatomical outlet obstruction secondary to prostatic enlarge-ment, where it has been reported to exist in up to 50% of patients (Hebjørn et al. 1976; Andersen 1976; Turner-Warwick 1979). Following relief of the outlet obstruction, the involuntary bladder activity ultimately disappears in 50% to 75% of the patients so affected. Those who doubt that inflammation or irritation at the level of the bladder itself can cause involuntary contractions during filling have only to observe the clinical occurrence of the symptoms of bladder 'spasm' secondary to catheter-induced irritation, and then observe their urodynamic correlate during filling. Decreased compliance during filling, which refers to a pathologically increased slope of the cystometric accommodation limb, may be secondary to the sequelae of neurological injury or disease, but may also result from a fixed small-capacity fibrotic bladder.

Although a number of factors seem to be involved in the genesis of classical stress urinary incontinence in the female, this seems primarily to be a sphincter dysfunction caused by a failure of the normal transmission of increases in intra-abdominal pressure to the proximal urethra (McGuire et al. 1976; McGuire 1979). This is felt to be due mainly to a change in the anatomical position of the vesico-urethral junction and proximal urethra which accompanies pelvic floor weakness or relaxation due to a number of causes. A deficient mucosal seal mechanism has also been postulated as a contributory factor in elderly hypo-oestrogenic women (Raz et al. 1973). Damage to the innervation of the smooth muscle of the bladder neck or proximal urethra, or to the periurethral striated muscle, may also result in a decrease in outlet resistance. Ageing, autonomic or somatic neuropathy, or surgical damage may be responsible for such pathology. Surgery or the ageing process may also have a direct adverse effect on the smooth musculature of the bladder neck and proximal urethra. Generally, these decreases in the factors which contribute to the outlet continence mechanisms are relative, and not an all-or-none phenomenon.

Urinary incontinence is a classical symptom of a failure of the bladder to fill and store urine adequately. Incontinence secondary to a fistula and so-called overflow or paradoxical incontinence are obvious exceptions. Urgency may be defined as the extreme desire to void, either because of pain or because of a fear of leaking urine. Urgency which is only pain-associated is generally secondary to inflammatory disease. Urodynamic measurements may be normal. Urgency associated with a fear of leaking urine, or a history of doing so, is generally associated with involuntary bladder contractions. An increase in daytime urinary frequency may simply be psychogenic in origin. However, it may be indicative of a genuine need to void, because of either pain or low-volume bladder distension, usually indicative of inflammatory disease, or from involuntary bladder contractions. Increased frequency may result also on a secondary basis from a failure to empty adequately, either because of a decreased functional bladder capacity or in assocation with detrusor hyperreflexia induced by outlet obstruction. Nocturia usually accompanies non-psychogenic urinary frequency.

The symptom of 'pressure' defies exact definition. It is not quite the urge to void but, in many people at least, there is the feeling that the bladder is full or that the urge to void will occur shortly. Often, no urodynamically discernible voiding dysfunction is found. However, the sensation of pressure can be due to a pathologically elevated intravesical pressure during filling, but one which is below that necessary to elicit the sensation of true distension or urgency.

Pharmacological treatment of abnormalities related to the filling–storage phase of micturition is conceptually simple. Therapy is directed towards inhibiting bladder contractility, or decreasing sensory input during filling, or towards increasing outlet resistance.

Pharmacotherapy to Decrease Bladder Contractility

Anticholinergic Agents

Atropine, and agents which imitate its action, produces a competitive blockade of acetylcholine receptors at postganglionic parasympathetic receptor sites. These agents have little effect at the level of autonomic ganglia (Innes and Nickerson 1975). Because at least a major portion of the neurohumoral stimulus for physiological bladder contraction is acetylcholine-induced stimulation of postganglionic parasympathetic cholinergic receptor sites on bladder smooth muscle, atropine and its cogeners will depress true involuntary contractions of any aetiology (Pederson and Grynderup 1966; Diokno et al. 1972; Innes and Nickerson 1975; Blaivas et al. 1980; Jensen 1981). In patients with detrusor hyperreflexia, the volume to the first involuntary contraction will generally be increased, the amplitude of the contractions decreased, and the total bladder capacity increased, with a proportionate reduction in symptomatology. Interestingly, bladder compliance in normal individuals and in those with detrusor hyperreflexia, where the initial slope of the filling curve on cystometry is normal prior to the involuntary contractions, does not seem to be significantly altered (Jensen 1981). The effect of these agents on intravesical pressure during filling in those patients who exhibit only decreased compliance has not been well studied.

In patients with detrusor hyperreflexia, although significant clinical improvement is achieved which is often acceptable to both patient and physician, only partial inhibition generally results. This is because of the phenomenon of atropine resistance, which refers to the ability of atropine to antagonise only partially the bladder response to neural or direct electrical stimulation, as opposed to its ability to block completely the response of bladder muscle strips to acetylcholine. The most attractive explanation for this phenomenon is that one or more non-cholinergic neurotransmitters are released, in addition to acetylcholine, by pelvic nerve stimulation (see Wein and Raezer 1979, for a complete discussion). The clinical correlate of this laboratory phenomenon is that it is rare to achieve a perfect result in the treatment of detrusor hyperreflexia with only an antimuscarinic agent or any single type of pharmacological treatment. Outlet resistance, reflected by intra-urethral pressure measurements, does not seem to be affected by anticholinergic therapy (Ulmsten et al. 1977). The potentially troublesome side-effects of all antimuscarinic agents include inhibition of salivary secretion (dry mouth), blockade of the iris sphincter muscle (pupillary dilation) and the lens ciliary muscle to cholinergic stimulation (blurred vision for near objects), tachycardia, drowsiness, and inhibition of gut motility (Weiner 1980a). Those agents which possess some ganglionic blocking activity may also cause orthostatic hypotension at high doses. Antimuscarinic agents are contraindicated in patients with narrow-angle glaucoma and should be used with caution in those with significant bladder outlet obstruction, as complete urinary retention may be precipitated.

Although atropine sulphate is available as a 0.5 mg tablet form, and it and all related anticholinergic agents are well absorbed from the gastro-intestinal tract, propantheline bromide (Pro-Banthine) is the oral agent which is most commonly used to produce an antimuscarinic effect in the lower urinary tract. The usual adult oral dosage is 15–30 mg every 4–6 hours. Oral administration in the fasting state rather than with or after meals is preferable from the standpoint of bioavailability (Gibaldi and Grundhofer 1975). The clinical efficacy can generally be predicted by observation of the effect of a parenteral dose on the cystometrogram (Blaivas et al. 1980). The parenteral preparation is no longer available, at least in many hospitals in the United States, and atropine or glycopyrrolate (Robinul) may be used instead. For such studies, we generally use 0.2 mg of glycopyrrolate (available as a 1 ml single-dose vial) (Mirakhur et al. 1978; Mirakhur and Dundee 1980). There seems to be little difference between the antimuscarinic effects on bladder smooth muscle of propantheline and those of other antimuscarinic agents such as glycopyrrolate (Robinul), isopropamide (Darbid), hyoscyamine (Cystospaz), and anisotropine methylbromide (Valpin). Some of these agents, such as glycopyrrolate, have a more convenient dosage schedule (twice or three times daily), but their clinical effects on the lower urinary tract seem to be indistinguishable.

Although there are obviously many other considerations which account for the activity of a given dose of drug as its site of action, there is no oral drug available whose direct antimuscarinic binding potential, at least in vitro, approximates that of atropine better than the long-available and relatively inexpensive propantheline bromide (Levin et al. 1982).

It would seem that an agent with a significant ganglionic blocking action as well as such action at the peripheral receptor level, might be more effective in suppressing bladder contractility. Although methantheline (Banthine) has a higher ratio of ganglionic blocking to antimuscarinic activity than does propantheline, the latter drug, clinical dose per dose, seems to be at least as potent in each respect (Weiner 1980a). Methantheline does have similar effects on the lower urinary tract, however, and some clinicians still prefer it, in doses of 50–100 mg four times a day, over other anticholinergic agents (Lapides and Dodson 1953; Hebjørn 1977).

Emepronium bromide (Cetiprin) is an anticholinergic agent which has been reported to have activity at both peripheral and ganglionic levels (Stanton 1973; Hebjørn and Walter 1978). It has been reported to increase bladder capacity in patients with detrusor hyperreflexia, while decreasing intravesical pressure and urinary flow (Ekeland and Sander 1976).

Recommended oral dosages range from 100 mg three times daily to 200 mg four times daily (Meyhoff and Nordling 1981). However, Ritch et al. (1977) failed to show any significant effect with oral therapy (200 mg three times daily), although they did demonstrate a good end-organ response with parenteral administration (50 mg intramuscularly). Cardozo and Stanton (1979) likewise found a clinically significant effect with a parenteral dose of 50 mg. Bladder responses to an intramuscular dose of 0.3 mg/kg, however, were found to be insignificant (Perera et al. 1982). In elderly patients with urinary incontinence and involuntary bladder contractions, Walter et al. (1982) found no difference between the effects of emepronium (200 mg three times daily) and a placebo, although there was a significant overall subjective cure or improvement rate of 79% in both groups. Potential side-effects of this agent are predominantly antimuscarinic, but they also include mucosal alteration, which sometimes leads to oral ulcers and oesophagitis. Emepronium is not available for use in the United States.

Musculotropic Relaxants (Antispasmodics)

Musculotropic relaxants come under the general heading of direct-acting smooth muscle depressants, whose 'antispasmodic' activity is reportedly directly on the smooth muscle at a site which is metabolically distal to the cholinergic receptor mechanism (Finkbeiner et al. 1978; Wein 1979). Although in the laboratory all three of the agents to be discussed do relax smooth muscle by a papaverine-like activity, all have been found to possess variable antimuscarinic and local anaesthetic properties. There is still some question as to how much of their clinical efficacy is due simply to their atropine-like effect. If any of these agents do in fact exert a clinically significant inhibitory effect which is independent of an antimuscarinic action, there does exist a therapeutic rationale for combining their use with that of a relatively pure antimuscarinic agent. It is certainly reasonable to try cautiously to combine pharmacological agents with different primary mechanisms of action (and hopefully different side-effects) in an attempt to achieve an additive clinical effect without a corresponding increase in the number or severity of side-effects.

Oxybutynin chloride (Ditropan) has been described as a moderately potent anticholinergic agent with strong independent musculotropic relaxant activity and local anaesthetic activity as well (Lish et al. 1965; Fredericks et al. 1978; Finkbeiner et al. 1978). It has been used successfully to relieve urinary discomfort and 'bladder spasm' following endoscopic resection (Diokno and Lapides 1972; Paulson 1978). A randomised double-blind control study comparing the effects of oxybutynin (5 mg three times daily) and a placebo in 30 patients with detrusor instability was carried out by Moisey et al. (1980). Seventeen of the 30 patients experienced side-effects with oxybutynin. Of 23 patients who completed the study with oxybutynin, 17 had symptomatic improvement and 9 had evidence of urodynamic improvement, mainly an increase in bladder volume at first contraction and an increase in total bladder capacity. The recommended adult dosage of oxybutynin is 5 mg three or four times daily. The potential side-effects are the same as those of propantheline.

Dicyclomine hydrochloride (Bentyl) is another agent reported to possess a direct relaxant effect on smooth muscle, in addition to an anticholinergic action (Johns et al. 1976; Downie et al. 1977; Khanna et al. 1979). An oral dose of 20 mg three times daily in adults has been reported to increase bladder capacity in patients with detrusor hyperreflexia (Fischer et al. 1978). Our own experience suggests that the individual dose must often be raised to at least 30 mg to achieve a good clinical effect. The potential side-effects are anticholinergic.

Flavoxate hydrochloride (Urispas) is another compound which has been reported to have a direct inhibitory action on smooth muscle, in addition to anticholinergic and local analgesic properties (Kohler and Morales 1968; Bradley and Cazort 1970). Favourable clinical effects have been noted in patients with frequency, urgency and incontinence, and in patients with urodynamically documented detrusor hyperreflexia (Stanton 1973; Delaere et al. 1977; Jonas et al. 1979b). However, Briggs et al. (1980) reported essentially no effect of this agent on detrusor hyperreflexia in an elderly population, an experience that would coincide with our own subjective impression of limited clinical efficacy in situations where other, less expensive agents have failed (Benson et al. 1977). The recommended adult dosage is 100–200 mg three or four times daily; as with all agents in this group, a short clinical trial may be worthwhile. Reported side-effects are rare and primarily anticholinergic.

Beta-Adrenergic Agonists

The presence of beta-adrenergic receptors in human bladder muscle has prompted attempts to increase bladder capacity with beta-adrenergic stimulation. Such stimulation can cause significant increases in the capacity of animal bladders which contain a moderate density of beta receptors (Larsen and Mortensen 1978). In vitro studies show a strong dose-related relaxant effect of beta-2 agonists on the bladder body of rabbits, but little effect on the bladder base or proximal urethra (Khanna et al. 1981). Terbutaline (Bricanyl) in oral dosages of 5 mg three times daily, has been reported to have a 'good clinical effect' in some patients with urgency and urgency incontinence, but no significant effect on the bladders of neurologically normal humans without voiding difficulty (Norlén et al. 1978). Although these results are compatible with those in other organ systems (beta-adrenergic stimulation causes no acute change in total lung capacity in normal humans while it does favourably affect patients with bronchial asthma), few if any adequate studies are available on the effects of beta-adrenergic stimulation in patients with detrusor hyperactivity.

Alpha-Adrenergic Antagonists

Jensen has reported an increased alpha-adrenergic effect in the bladders of patients he characterised as uninhibited (1981). Short-term and long-term administration of prazosin have been reported by him to increase bladder capacity and decrease the amplitude of contractions in this category of patient (1981). Rohner et al. (1978) found a change in the normal beta response of canine bladder body to an alpha response after bladder outlet obstruction. Perlberg and Caine (1982) studied the in vitro response of bladder dome muscle from patients with obstructive prostatic hypertrophy and found an alpha-adrenergic response to noradrenaline (instead of the usual beta response) in 23% of 47 patients. They speculated as to a potential relationship between irritative symptoms in these patients and this altered adrenergic response. They further theorised that at least some of the symptomatic improvement in irritative symptoms seen in patients with benign prostatic hypertrophy treated with alpha-adrenergic blocking agents may be due to a direct effect of these agents on bladder muscle, rather than their effect on outflow resistance. Although highly speculative, this potential avenue of therapy seems worthy of further study, though it should be noted that considerable improvement was obtained also with a placebo.

Prostaglandin Inhibitors

As mentioned previously, prostaglandins are one class of compound with a potentially important role in excitatory neurotransmission in the lower urinary tract. Recent experiments have suggested that they may contribute to purinergic excitation of rabbit and guinea-pig bladder smooth mucle (Andersson et al. 1980; Anderson 1982). Thus, there exist multiple mechanisms whereby inhibitors of prostaglandin synthesis might decrease bladder contractility.

Cardozo et al. (1980) reported such effects in a double-blind placebo study of 30 women with detrusor instability, in which they used the prostaglandin synthetase inhibitor flurbiprofen at a dosage of 50 mg three times daily. Abnormal bladder activity, however, was not abolished in significantly more drug-treated than placebo-treated patients, and actual bladder capacity likewise showed no change. It was concluded that the drug did not abolish detrusor hyperreflexia, but delayed the intravesical pressure rise to a greater level of distension. Forty-three per cent of the patients experienced side-effects from the drug, primarily nausea, vomiting, headache, indigestion, gastric distress, constipation and rash. Cardozo and Stanton (1980) reported symptomatic improvement in patients with detrusor instability given indomethacin, another prostaglandin synthetase inhibitor, in dosages of 50–200 mg daily. This was a short-term study with no cystometric data, and the drug was compared only with bromocriptine. The incidence of side-effects was high, although no patient had to stop treatment because of these. It is interesting that this category of agents has proved to be useful in primary dysmenorrhoea, a condition felt to be related to a high level of menstrual endometrial prostaglandin synthesis (Chan et al. 1981). Numerous prostaglandin inhibitors exist, most of which fall under the heading of non-steroidal anti-inflammatory drugs. The most common such agent, aspirin, is only a relatively weak inhibitor of prostaglandin synthesis.

Calcium Antagonists

The rationale underlying the potential use of calcium antagonists for the inhibition of bladder contractility has been described previously (see Chap. 2). The calcium antagonist nifedipine has been shown to be an effective inhibitor of contraction induced by several mechanisms in human and guinea-pig bladder muscle (Forman et al. 1978; Sjögren and Andersson 1979). It is capable also of completely blocking the non-cholinergic portion of the contraction produced by electrical field stimulation in rabbit bladder (Husted, Sjögren and Andersson, cited by Husted et al. 1980). Nifedipine more effectively inhibited potassium-induced than carbachol-induced contractions in bladder strips, whereas terodiline, an agent with both calcium antagonistic and anticholinergic properties, had the opposite effect (Husted et al. 1980). However, terodiline caused a complete inhibition of the response of rabbit bladder to electrical field stimulation. This agent in low concentrations seemed to have mainly an antimuscarinic action, whereas at higher concentrations a calcium antagonistic effect became evident. In vitro experiments appeared to show that these two effects are at least additive with regard to bladder contractility. Whether the calcium antagonistic properties of terodiline contribute to its clinical effectiveness in vivo, and whether the drug is actually more effective than standard antimuscarinic agents alone, remain to be established. Rud et al. (1980) reported that in oral dosages of 12.5 mg two or three times daily it produced a marked decrease in the number of hyperreflexic contractions in a group of 7 women with urgency incontinence and 2 with nocturnal enuresis. Bladder capacity was approximately doubled, and the amplitude of the contractions was decreased. In a double-blind cross-over study in 12 women with motor urge incontinence, Ekman et al. (1980) reported an increase in bladder capacity and in the volume at which the sensation of urgency was experienced in all but one of the patients treated with terodiline, whereas placebo treatment had no effect on either objective or subjective parameters.

Palmer et al. (1981) reported a double-blind placebo trial with a single 20 mg daily dose of flunarizine in 14 females with urinary frequency, incontinence, and urodynamically proven detrusor instability. A statistically significant decrease in urgency was produced in the flunarizine-treated group, but there was no change in the frequency of micturition. Although there was a trend towards improvement of cystometric parameters, this was not statistically significant at the $P = 0.05$ level. The side-effects produced in patients who have been treated with calcium antagonists for voiding dysfunction have been small in number, but it should be noted that the potential side-effects of these agents can be considerable and consist of hypotension, facial flushing, headache, dizziness, abdominal discomfort, constipation, nausea, skin rash, weakness and palpitations. Although work in this area is obviously in its infancy, this class of agents may yet prove to be a promising alternative or addition to existing treatment for the inhibition of bladder contractility.

Dimethyl Sulphoxide (DMSO)

Dimethyl sulphoxide (DMSO) is a relatively simple naturally occurring organic compound which has been used as an industrial solvent for many years. Among its properties is its ability to penetrate the intact skin, transporting chemicals along with it for absorption into the bloodstream. It has multiple pharmacological actions (membrane penetrant, anti-inflammatory, local analgesic, bacteriostatic, diuretic, cholinesterase inhibitor, collagen solvent, vasodilatory) and is used for the treatment of arthritis and other musculoskeletal disorders (*Medical Letter* 1980; Council on Scientific Affairs (AMA) 1982). The only formulation approved for use on human bladder is a 50% solution; a 70% solution is generally used topically for musculoskeletal disorders.

Stewart and Shirley (1976) reported symptomatic improvement in 75% of patients with interstitial cystitis following a course of treatment with this agent, and an improvement in bladder capacity in 80% of these patients. Generally, one 50 ml intravesical instillation is carried out every other week for a total of six treatments. The solution is allowed to remain in the bladder for 15 minutes, after which it is expelled by spontaneous voiding. Fowler (1981) reported results with DMSO in 20 patients with early interstitial cystitis: 3 complete and 16 partial symptomatic remissions were achieved. However, functional bladder capacity, measured at the termination of therapy in 18 cases, was observed to increase by more than 25% in only 4 patients. In 10 patients with severe detrusor hyperreflexia, Andersen et al. (1981) were able to demonstrate no subjective or objective effects of the drug. The unpleasant garlic-type odour of DMSO is its primary side-effect and makes double-blind placebo studies impossible. Cataracts have been reported in experimental animals but not in humans; eye evaluation is, however, recommended with chronic therapy. As a last resort, this drug has been used by some clinicians in the frustrating patient with the urgency–frequency syndrome but without objective evidence of true interstitial cystitis or detrusor hyperreflexia. Although anecdotal improvement is sometimes reported few, if any, formal reports of the results of such therapy exist.

Urgency–Frequency Incontinence Without Involuntary Bladder Contraction

It is obvious that there are a number of patients who have symptoms which suggest detrusor hyperreflexia or instability but who in fact have no detectable consistent abnormalities during the filling phase of micturition. Most of these patients report symptoms of urgency, frequency, dysuria, pressure and incontinence in varying proportions. The treatment of this symptom complex is, initially at least, usually empirical and consists of one or a combination of the agents discussed here under the category of 'Pharmacotherapy to Decrease Bladder Contractility'. The fact that most of these patients do not have involuntary bladder contractions most probably accounts for the generally less than optimal results achieved with this type of treatment (Rees et al. 1976; Ulmsten et al. 1977). Urodynamic evaluation of these patients may show variations in urethral pressures, or may be entirely normal. Whether attempts at pharmacological correction of these urethral urodynamic abnormalities would significantly alter symptomatology is as yet unknown. Fossberg et al. (1981) did report successful subjective results with phenylpropanolamine (50 mg twice daily) in 22 of 34 female patients with sensory urge incontinence, many of whom had wide urethral pressure variations during filling.

It should seem that the ideal pharmacological treatment for at least the urgency, frequency and dysuria component of this symptom complex, which seems to be more sensory than motor in origin, would be an agent which produces topical anaesthesia or hypoesthaesia of the bladder and urethral mucosa. Although there are agents, such as Pyridium, which are reported to have this action as their primary effect, the clinical results which have been obtained with such compounds in these circumstances, at least by us, have been poor. There is no doubt that, in at least some of these patients, the symptoms exist only on a psychosomatic basis. However, in many there may in fact exist an as yet undetected abnormality, or various categories of abnormalities, which may ultimately prove susceptible to pharmacological management.

Pharmacotherapy to Increase Outlet Resistance

Alpha-Adrenergic Agonists

Various orally administered pharmacological agents are available to produce alpha-adrenergic stimulation with relatively mild side-effects. As the smooth muscle of the outlet contains abundant alpha receptor sites, one would expect outlet resistance to be increased by such an action. Potential side-effects of all of these agents include blood pressure elevation, anxiety and insomnia due to stimulation of the central nervous system. They also may cause headache, tremor, weakness, dizziness, respiratory difficulties, palpitations and cardiac arrythmias. All should be used with caution in patients with hypertension, cardiovascular disease or hyperthyroidism (Weiner 1980b).

Ephedrine is a non-catecholamine sympathomimetic agent which owes part of its peripheral action to the release of noradrenaline, but which also directly stimulates both alpha- and beta-adrenergic receptors (Weiner 1980b). The oral adult dosage is 25–50 mg four times daily. Some tachyphylaxis develops to its peripheral actions, probably as a result of depletion of noradrenaline stores. Pseudoephedrine (Sudafed) is a stereoisomer of ephedrine which is used for similar indications with similar precautions (Wein 1979). The adult dosage is 30–60 mg four times daily, and the 30 mg dose form is available in the United States without a prescription. The use of ephedrine for stress urinary incontinence was mentioned as early as 1948, by Rashbaum and Mandelbaum.

Acutely, norephedrine chloride in a dose of 75–100 mg was shown to increase maximal urethral pressure and maximal urethral closure pressure in women with urinary stress incontinence (Ek et al. 1978). At a 300 ml bladder volume, the maximal urethral pressure rose from 82 to 110 cm of water and the maximal urethral closure pressure rose from 63 to 93 cm of water. The functional profile length did not change significantly. A 14-day double-blind cross-over study comparing the effects of norephedrine with a placebo showed that reduction of urinary leakage with the drug as compared with a placebo occurred in 12 of 22 patients. The maximal urethral pressure and maximal urethral closure pressure were increased over those with a placebo by only 10% and 14% respectively, however. Diokno and Taub (1975) reported a good to excellent response in 27 of 38 patients with sphincteric incontinence treated with ephedrine sulphate. They noted that beneficial effects were most often achieved in those with minimal to moderate wetting, and that little benefit was achieved in those patients with severe stress incontinence. Öbrink and Bunne (1978) noted that 100 mg of norephedrine chloride twice daily did not improve the severe stress incontinence of 10 female patients sufficiently to offer an alternative to surgical treatment. They further noted in this group that the maximal urethral closure pressure was not influenced at rest or with stress at low or moderate bladder volumes.

Phenylpropanolamine hydrochloride (Propadrine) shares the pharmacological properties of ephedrine and is approximately equal in peripheral potency, while causing less central stimulation (Weiner 1980b). Using a dosage of 50 mg three times daily, Awad et al. (1978) found that, after 4 weeks of therapy the stress incontinence (severity not noted) of 11 of 13 females and 6 of 7 males was significantly improved. Maximal urethral closure pressure was increased from a mean of 47 cm of water to 72 in the empty bladder and from 43 to 58 cm of water with a full bladder. The preparation used was 50 mg of phenylpropranolamine combined with 8 mg of chlorpheniramine (an antihistamine) and 2.5 mg of isopropamide (an antimuscarinic) as a sustained-release capsule called Ornade, which is used primarily for the relief of symptoms of allergic rhinitis. Using one capsule twice daily, Stewart et al. (1976) found that, of 77 female patients with urinary stress incontinence, 18 were completely cured, 28 were much better, 6 were slightly better, and 25 were no better. In 11 patients with post-prostatectomy stress incontinence, the numbers in the corresponding categories were 1, 2, 1 and 7. Subsequently, Montague and Stewart (1979) carried out urethral profilometry in 12 females with moderate to marked stress incontinence and 6 with no history of incontinence. The maximal urethral pressure increased by more than 20% in 11 of the incontinent patients and only 1 in the continent group.

Rees and Ransley (1980) reported on the use of Ornade in 83 children with daytime wetting from a variety of causes. Of 24 children with bladder neck incompetence, 41% were cured, 29% had minimal symptoms and 12% were improved. Interestingly, of 31 patients with bladder instability, the corresponding percentages were 24, 24 and 20. This latter beneficial effect may have been due to the anticholinergic agent in the preparation. Treatment had to be stopped in 8 children because of side-effects; 23 other children had mild and transient side-effects. Major surgery was avoided by drug treatment in 4 children. The formulation of Ornade has now been changed, such that each capsule contains 75 mg of phenylpropanolamine and 12 mg of chlorpheniramine. It is also available as a liquid.

Midodrin is a long-acting alpha-adrenergic stimulator reported to be useful in the treatment of seminal emission and ejaculation disorders following retro-peritoneal lymphadenectomy (Jonas et al. 1979a). Treatment with 5 mg twice daily for 4 weeks in 20 females with stress incontinence produced a cure in 1 and improvement in 14 (Kiesswetter et al. 1983). The mean maximal urethral closure pressure rose by 8.3% and the planimetric index of the continence area on profilometry increased by 9%. This agent is not yet available for general use in the United States.

Although spectacular cure and improvement rates have been reported with alpha-adrenergic agonists in females with stress urinary incontinence, our own experience coincides with that of authors who report that stimulation with such agents often produces improvement but rarely produces total dryness in cases of severe or even moderate stress incontinence. A clinical trial is certainly worthwhile, however, and will, at the least, assure the patient that the possibility of one type of non-surgical therapy has been explored.

Beta-Adrenergic Antagonists

Theoretically, beta-adrenergic blocking agents might be expected to 'unmask' or potentiate an alpha-adrenergic effect, thereby increasing outlet resistance. Gleason et al. (1974) reported success in treating certain patients with stress urinary incontinence with propranolol, a beta-adrenergic blocking agent, with oral dosages of 10 mg four times daily. The beneficial effect, however, became manifest only after 4–10 weeks of treatment, a fact which is difficult to explain on a pharmacological basis, as the cardiac effects occur rather promptly after administration. However, the hypotensive effects of propranolol do not usually appear as rapidly (Weiner 1980c). Such treatment has been suggested as an alternative method (to alpha-adrenergic stimulation) of pharmacological therapy in patients with hypertension and stress incontinence. Few, if any, subsequent reports have appeared to support this approach, and it should be noted that others have been unable to show significant increases in urethral profilometry pressures in normal females after administration of a beta-adrenergic blocking agent (Donker and Van der Sluis 1976). Although 10 mg four times daily is a relatively small dosage of propranolol, it should be remembered that the major potential side-effects are related to the drug's therapeutic beta-adrenergic blocking effects. Heart failure may develop, as well as an increase in airway resistance, and asthma is a contraindication to the use of this drug. Administration of any beta-adrenergic blocking agent, in addition, renders patients suscept-ible to a withdrawal syndrome that is probably due to supersensitivity of beta-adrenergic receptors (Weiner 1980c). Abrupt discontinuation may precipitate an exacerbation of anginal attacks and rebound hypertension.

The Effect of Imipramine on the Lower Urinary Tract

Some authors have found tricyclic antidepressants, particularly imipramine hydrochloride (Tofranil, SK-Pramine, Janimine) to be particularly useful for facilitating urinary storage (Milner and Hills 1968; Petersen et al. 1974; Raezer et al. 1977; Castleden et al. 1981). These agents have been the subject of a voluminous amount of highly sophisticated pharmacological investigation to determine the mechanisms of action responsible for their varied effects

(Hollister 1978; Rosenbaum et al. 1979; Baldessarini 1980; Richelson 1983). Most of the investigations have had the aim of explaining their antidepressant properties, and consequently have been carried out primarily on central nervous system tissue. The results and the conclusions and speculations inferred from them, are extremely interesting, but it must be emphasised that it is essentially unknown whether they apply to or have relevance for the lower urinary tract.

All of these agents possess varying degrees of at least three major pharmacological actions: they have central and peripheral anticholinergic actions at some, but not all, sites; they block the active transport system in the presynaptic nerve ending which is responsible for the re-uptake of the released amine neurotransmitters serotonin and noradrenaline; and they are sedatives, an action which occurs presumably on a central basis but is perhaps related to their antihistaminic properties. There is also evidence that they desensitise alpha-2 receptors on central noradrenergic neurons (Crews and Smith 1978; Spyraki and Fibiger 1980). Paradoxically, they have also been shown to block alpha-1 adrenergic receptors and serotonin receptors. Many such compounds are available and have been categorised as to their relative potency insofar as their multiple effects are concerned.

Imipramine has prominent systemic anticholinergic effects (Baldessarini 1980). However, it appears to have only a weak antimuscarinic effect on bladder smooth muscle (Diokno et al. 1972; Dhattiwala 1976; Olubadewo 1980), similar to its effect on salivary gland function (Tulloch and Creed 1979). A strong direct inhibitory effect on bladder smooth muscle does exist, however, which is neither anticholinergic nor adrenergic (Dhattiwala 1976; Benson et al. 1977; Fredericks et al. 1978; Tulloch and Creed 1979; Olubadewo 1980). This may be due to a local-anaesthetic-like action at the nerve terminals in the adjacent effector membrane, an effect that seems to occur also in cardiac muscle (Bigger et al. 1977), or to an inhibition of the participation of calcium in the excitation–contraction coupling process (Olubadewo 1980). Clinically, the drug seems effective in decreasing bladder contractility and in increasing outlet resistance (Cole and Fried 1972; Mahony et al. 1973; Raezer et al. 1977; Tulloch and Creed 1979; Castleden et al. 1981). Trying to correlate mechanism of action with clinical effect, one might postulate that the increase in outlet resistance is due to a peripheral blockade of noradrenaline re-uptake, which would tend to produce or enhance an alpha-adrenergic effect in the smooth muscle of the bladder base and proximal urethra. Theoretically at least, this latter action, if indeed it occurs in the lower urinary tract as it does centrally, might tend also to stimulate predominantly beta-adrenergic receptors in bladder body smooth musculature, an action which would further facilitate urine storage by decreasing the excitability of smooth muscle in that area.

Castleden et al. (1981) began therapy in elderly patients with detrusor instability with a single 25 mg night-time dose which was increased every third day by 25 mg until either the patient was continent or had side-effects, or a dose of 150 mg was reached. Six of 10 patients became continent and, in those who underwent repeat cystometry, bladder capacity increased by a mean of 105 ml and bladder pressure at capacity decreased by a mean of 18 cm of water. Maximal urethral pressure increased by a mean of 30 cm of water. Although our subjective impression (Raezer et al. 1977) was that such effects became evident only after days of treatment, some patients in this series became continent after only 3–5 days of treatment. Our usual adult dosage of imipramine for voiding dysfunction is 25 mg four times daily, and half that dose in elderly patients. In our experience the effects of imipramine on the lower urinary tract are often additive to those of the atropine-like agents. Consequently, a combination of imipramine and propantheline is sometimes especially useful for decreasing bladder contractility (Raezer et al. 1977). If imipramine is to be used in conjunction with an atropine-like agent, it should be noted that the anticholinergic side-effects of the drugs may be additive.

It has been known for many years that imipramine is relatively effective in the treatment of childhood nocturnal enuresis (Noack 1964; Woodhead et al. 1967; Kunin et al. 1970). Dosages have ranged from 10 mg daily to 50 mg daily. Whether the mechanism of action is the same as that of imipramine in decreasing bladder contractility or increasing outlet resistance, or whether it is centrally mediated, is unknown. Korczyn and Kish (1979) have presented evidence that the anti-enuretic effect is neither on a peripheral anticholinergic basis nor on the same basis as whatever effects are responsible for the drug's antidepressant action. The anti-enuretic effect occurs soon after initial administration, whereas the antidepressant effects generally take 2–4 weeks to develop.

When used in the generally larger doses employed for antidepressant effects, the most frequent side-effects of this group of agents are those attributable to their systemic anticholinergic activity. Allergic phenomena, including rash, elevated liver function, obstructive jaundice and agranulocytosis may also occur, but rarely. Side-effects on the central nervous system may include weakness, fatigue, a parkinsonian effect, a fine tremor most noted in the upper extremities, and a manic or schizophrenic picture. Sedation may also result from an antihistaminic effect. Postural hypotension may be seen, presumably on the basis of alpha-1 receptor blockade.

Antidepressants can be shown electrophysiologically and haemodynamically to have a depressant effect upon the myocardium shortly after their institution (Burgess and Turner 1980; Muller and Schulze 1980). However, Veith et al. (1982) have pointed out that, in the animal studies showing a direct myocardial depressant effect, this occurs at plasma concentrations which are in the toxic range for humans. This group of investigators followed 24 depressed patients with heart disease treated for 4 weeks and found that tricyclic antidepressants had no effect on left ventricular ejection fraction at rest or during maximal exercise. The mean daily dose of imipramine in their series was 129 mg, and they suggest that such antidepressant doses can be used in depressed patients with pre-existing heart disease, except for those with severely impaired myocardial performance, without an adverse effect on ventricular rhythm or haemodynamic function. Whether cardiotoxicity will prove to be a legitimate concern in patients receiving somewhat smaller doses for lower urinary tract dysfunction remains to be seen, and is a potential matter of concern.

If imipramine or any of the tricyclic antidepressants is to be prescribed for the treatment of voiding dysfunction, the patient should be thoroughly informed of the usual indications, the potential side-effects, and, in the United States, of the fact that this drug is not approved by the Federal Regulatory Agency for this purpose. The onset of significant side-effects (severe abdominal distress, nausea, vomiting, headache, lethargy and irritability) following abrupt cessation of high doses of imipramine in children (Petti and Law 1981), would suggest that the drug should be discontinued gradually, especially in patients receiving high doses. Tricyclic antidepressants can also cause excess sweating of obscure aetiology and a delay of orgasm and orgasmic impotence, whose cause is likewise unclear (Baldessarini 1980). The use of imipramine is contraindicated in patients receiving monoamine oxidase inhibitors, as severe central nervous system toxicity (hyperpyrexia, seizures and coma) can be precipitated.

Oestrogen Therapy

Salmon, Walter and Geist first reported the use of oestrogen in the treatment of stress urinary incontinence in 1941. Raz et al. (1973) found that a daily dose of 2.5 mg of Premarin improved stress incontinence and increased urethral pressures in post-menopausal patients, effects which they attributed to mucosal proliferation with a consequently improved 'mucosal seal effect' and to enhancement of the alpha-adrenergic contractile response of urethral smooth musculature to endogenous catecholamines. Schreiter et al. (1976) reported similar benefits after 10 days of treatment with daily divided doses of 6 mg of oestriol. They showed also that the effects of oestrogen and of exogenous alpha-adrenergic stimulation were additive. Hodgson et al. (1978) reported that the sensitivity of the rabbit urethra to alpha-adrenergic stimulation was oestrogen dependent, as castration caused a decreased sensitivity, and treatment with low levels of oestrogen reversed the defect.

Rud (1980a) studied the effects of 4 mg daily doses of oestradiol and 8 mg daily doses of oestriol on 30 females with an average age of 61 years, 24 of whom had stress urinary incontinence. Profilometry parameters were recorded at a bladder volume of 200 ml using microtransducer technique. Small but statistically significant changes occurred in the maximal urethral pressure (59 to 63 cm of water), functional urethral length (25 to 28 mm) and actual urethral length (33 to 37 mm). No statistically significant change occurred in urethral closure pressure (37 to 39 cm of water). Eight of the 24 incontinent patients experienced subjective and objective improvement, 9 experienced subjective improvement only, and 7 experienced neither subjective nor objective improvement. There was no correlation between subjective or objective improvement and the previously mentioned urodynamic measurements. However, in 18 patients pressure transmission to the urethra was recorded during cough, and in 7 of these this improved. All of these had subjective improvement and 5 were shown to be objectively dry. Rud himself points out that it is hard to believe that the small changes in urodynamic measurements, even though statistically significant, are directly related to resumption of continence. He noted also that the increased pressure transmission ratio might be due to factors outside the urethra—either in the striated musculature of the pelvic floor or in the peri-urethral vasculature or supporting tissues. Interestingly, he found no changes in urodynamic measurements in 5 continent and 3 stress incontinent females with cystic glandular hyperplasia treated with a single injection of 1000 mg of intramuscular progesterone, except that the pressure transmission ratio was lower in the 3 patients in whom this was measured.

Rud (1980b) also studied profilomety during the menstrual cycle in 6 females. There was no change in any profilometric values during the menstrual cycle and no correlation between oestrogen levels and maximal urethral pressure. It may be, as he suggests, that at physiological levels oestrogens have little influence on urodynamic measurements related to continence, and that only pharmacological doses cause urodynamically significant changes; further, pharmacological doses may alter responses to other exogenous autonomic stimulation, particularly alpha-adrenergic, as the previously described laboratory experiments by Hodgson et al. (1978) would suggest.

Beisland et al. (1981) administered 80 mg of oestriol intramuscularly every 4 weeks in combination with an oral dosage of phenylpropanolamine of 50 mg twice daily to a group of 13 patients with what they described as an incompetent urethral closure mechanism, that is, proximal sphincter hypofunction. Patients with genuine stress incontinence were excluded. These patients had a poor urethral pressure profile and a low maximal urethral closure pressure. All patients, however, had adequate transmission of increased abdominal pressure to the bladder and to the urethra. Eight of these patients became continent, and 4 showed improvement. The average maximal urethral closure pressure increased from 24.6 to 43.6 cm of water ($P > 0.005$). In the one patient in whom maximal urethral closure pressure did not change, the clinical condition likewise was unchanged.

Recent experiments (Levin et al. 1980, 1981) have shown that parenteral oestrogen administration can change the alpha-adrenergic receptor content and the autonomic innervation of the lower urinary tract of immature female rabbits. Whether these experiments have any clinical significance is unknown. Certainly, oestrogen therapy seems capable of facilitating urinary storage in some female patients by increasing outlet resistance, and there is evidence of an augmentative or perhaps additive effect with alpha-adrenergic therapy in this regard. Whether the levels achieved by the commonly used oral or parenteral oestrogen preparations or by oestrogen vaginal creams (which simply provide a convenient vehicle for systemic absorption) actually increase the alpha-adrenergic receptor content of the smooth muscle of the bladder outlet or the 'mucosal seal effect' is still a matter for speculation and is currently under study.

The potential long-term effects of such treatment must be carefully considered, however, in the light of the current controversy over whether oestrogen therapy predisposes to the development of endometrial carcinoma. At the very least, if a beneficial effect on the lower urinary tract is achieved by a regimen which uses oestrogenic therapy alone or in combination with other therapy, the lowest maintenance dose of oestrogen therapy possible should ultimately be used, one which it is to be hoped is below that used for replacement therapy in menopausal and post-menopausal women.

Antidiuretic-Hormone-Like Agents

A novel approach to the treatment of urinary frequency occurring within a specific period of time has been the use of synthetic antidiuretic hormone (vasopressin) analogues. DDAVP (desmopressin acetate) has been used effectively in patients with central diabetes insipidus to increase the osmolality of urine and decrease its volume (intranasal spray administration of 5–20 µg produced 8–20 hours of antidiuresis in 8 patients with central diabetes insipidus: Robinson 1976). The drug is well tolerated in both adults and children (Kosman 1978). For diabetes insipidus, the usual adult dosage is 0.01–0.04 mg daily as a single or divided dose. (DDAVP has a much greater antidiuretic potency than lysine or arginine vasopressin, a more prolonged duration of action (generally

8–10 hours), and virtually no pressor activity.) For children, the usual dosage range is from 0.005 to 0.03 mg daily. Large doses may cause transient headaches, nausea and a slight increase in blood pressure. Fluid intake should be adjusted during this therapy to avoid hyponatraemia and water intoxication.

The drug has been used to decrease the frequency of nocturnal enuresis. In one study of 22 children the number of wet nights per 2 weeks for desmopressin-treated children was 4.2 compared with 10.9 for those given a placebo. In 19 of 22 patients the response during DDAVP therapy was better than that during placebo (Birkásová et al. 1978). A single night-time dose of 10–40 µg was used. Ramsden et al. (1982) completed a double-blind cross-over trial of DDAVP and a placebo in 21 adult patients with nocturnal enuresis who were wet more than 20 nights per month. The total number of nights wet on the active drug was statistically less than that on placebo (91 vs. 167). Sixteen patients had fewer nights wet on treatment with active drug, 2 on placebo, and 3 showed no difference. Eight patients on the active drug became entirely dry or had only one night wet, compared with only 1 patient on placebo. The authors noted that 3 patients who had been taking active drug remained entirely dry. The dosage used was 20 mg intranasally at bedtime. Side-effects were few and minor.

Hilton and Stanton (1982) used a night-time dose of 20 mg intranasally in a double-blind placebo study of 25 female patients with nocturnal urinary frequency. The number of mean episodes per night decreased from 3.17 in the pretreatment group to 1.94 in the group treated with active drug, as compared with 2.61 in the placebo-treated group. The nocturnal urinary output, as expected, also decreased significantly in the drug-treated group. One patient, already on treatment for hypertension with a diuretic, became hypertensive with a diastolic pressure of 110 mm of mercury (entrance pressure was 80 mm of mercury). The authors emphasise that hypertension, ischaemic heart disease and congestive failure should all be considered contraindications to the use of this type of medication. A double-blind placebo-controlled study was also carried out in a group of 21 males with benign prostatic hypertrophy and significant nocturia (Månsson et al. 1980). Active treatment consisted of 20 mg of drug administered intranasally. This produced a mean fall in nocturia from 2.60 episodes during the control period to 1.93, statistically significantly better than the response to placebo (2.31) but hardly a significant clinical change.

Although the overall results with this type of agent in patients other than those with central diabetes insipidus seem more statistically than clinically significant, this class of treatment may prove to be useful on a long-term basis in the occasional case of nocturia or enuresis that has proved refractory to all other forms of therapy, or in acute situations where a decrease in intravesical volume and consequent urinary frequency is desired for a limited period of time.

This work was supported in part by a merit review grant from the Veterans Administration.

References

Abel BJ, Jameson RM, Gibbon NOK, Krishnan KR (1974) The neuropathic urethra. Lancet
    II:1229–1230
Abromowicz A (ed) (1978) Baclofen (Lioresal). Med Lett Drugs Ther 20:43–44
Allen TD (1977) The non-neurogenic neurogenic bladder. J Urol 117:232–238
Andersen JT (1976) Detrusor hyperreflexia in benign infravesical obstruction: a cystometric study.
    J Urol 115:532–534
Andersen JT, Walter S, Vejlsgaard R (1981) A clinical and bacteriological trial with DMSO in the
    treatment of severe detrusor hyperreflexia. Scand J Urol Nephrol [Suppl] 60:63–65
Anderson (1982) Evidence for a prostaglandin link in the purinergic activation of rabbit bladder
    smooth muscle. J Pharmacol Exp Ther 220: 347–352
Andersson K-E, Hustad S, Sjögren C (1980) Contribution of prostaglandins to the adenosine
    triphosphate induced contraction of rabbit urinary bladder. Br J Pharmacol 70: 443–452
Andersson K-E, Ek A, Hedlund H, Mattiasson A (1981) Effects of prazosin on isolated human
    urethra and in patients with lower motor neuron lesions. Invest Urol 19:39–42
Atkins FL, Nicolosi GL (1979) Alpha adrenergic blocking activity of prazosin. Biochem Pharmacol
    28:1233–1237
Awad SA, Downie JW, Kiruluta HG (1978) Alpha-adrenergic agents in urinary disorders of the
    proximal urethra. I. Sphincteric incontinence. Br J Urol 50:332–335
Baldessarini RJ (1980) Drugs and the treatment of psychiatric disorders. In: Gilman AG, Goodman
    LS, Gilman A (eds) The pharmacological basis of therapeutics. Macmillan, New York, pp
    391–447
Barrett DM (1981) The effect of oral bethanechol chloride on voiding in female patients with
    excessive residual urine: a randomized double-blind study. J Urol 126:640–642
Beisland HO, Fossberg E, Sander S (1981) On incompetent urethral closure mechanism: treatment
    with estriol and phenylpropanolamine. Scand J Urol Nephrol [Suppl] 60:67–69
Benson H, Epstein MD (1975) The placebo effect. JAMA 232:1225–1226
Benson GS, Sarshik SA, Raezer DM, Wein AJ (1977) Bladder muscle contractility: comparative
    effects and mechanisms of action of atropine, propantheline, flavoxate, and imipramine. Urology
    9:31–35
Bigger JT, Giardina EGV, Perel JM, Kantor SJ, Glassman AH (1977) Cardiac anti-arrhythmic
    effect of imipramine hydrochloride. N Engl J Med 296:206–208
Birkásová M, Birkás O, Flynn MJ, Cort JH (1978) Desmopressin in the management of nocturnal
    enuresis in children: a double-blind study. Pediatrics 62:970–974
Blaivas JG, Labib KB, Michalik SJ, Zayed AAH (1980) Cystometric response to propantheline in
    detrusor hyperreflexia: therapeutic implications. J Urol 124:259–262
Blaschke TF, Melmon KL (1980) Antihypertensive agents and drug therapy of hypertension. In:
    Gilman AG, Goodman LS, Gilman A (eds) The pharmacological basis of therapeutics.
    Macmillan, New York, pp 793–818
Bradley DV, Cazort RJ (1970) Relief of bladder spasm by flavoxate: a comparative study. J Clin
    Pharmacol 10:65–68
Briggs RS, Castleden CM, Asher MJ (1980) The effect of flavoxate on uninhibited detrusor
    contractions and urinary incontinence in the elderly. J Urol 123:665–666
Bultitude MI, Hills NH, Shuttleworth KED (1976) Clinical and experimental studies on the action
    of prostaglandins and their synthesis inhibitors on detrusor muscle in vitro and in vivo. Br J
    Urol 48:631–637
Burgess CD, Turner P (1980) Cardiotoxicity of antidepressant drugs. Neuropharmacology 19:
    1195–1199
Byck R (1975) Drugs and the treatment of psychiatric disorders. In: Goodman LS, Gilman A (eds)
    The pharmacological basis of therapeutics, 5th edn. Macmillan, New York, pp 152–200
Cameron MD (1966) Distigmine bromide (Ubretid) in the prevention of post-operative retention
    of urine. J Obstet Gynaecol Br Cwlth 73:847–848
Cardozo DL, Stanton SL (1979) An objective comparison of the effects of parenterally administered
    drugs in patients suffering from detrusor instability. J Urol 122:58–59
Cardozo LD, Stanton SL (1980) A comparison between bromocriptine and indomethacin in the
    treatment of detrusor instability. J Urol 123:399–401
Cardozo LD, Stanton SL, Robinson H, Hole D (1980) Evaluation of flurbiprofen in detrusor
    instability. Br Med J 280:281–282

Castleden CM, George CF, Renwick AG, Asher MJ (1981) Imipramine – a possible alternative to current therapy for urinary incontinence in the elderly. J Urol 125:318–320

Chan WY, Dawood MY, Fuchs F (1981) Prostaglandins in primary dysmenorrhea. Am J Med 70:535–541

Cole AT, Fried FA (1972) Favorable experiences with imipramine in the treatment of neurogenic bladder. J Urol 107:44–45

Council on Scientific Affairs, AMA (1982) Dimethyl sulfoxide. JAMA 248:1369–1371

Crews FT, Smith CB (1978) Presynaptic alpha receptor subsensitivity after long-term antidepressant treatment. Science 202:322–324

de Groat WC, Booth AM (1980) Physiology of the urinary bladder and urethra. Ann Int Med 92(2):312–315

de Groat WC, Saum WR (1972) Sympathetic inhibition of the urinary bladder and of pelvic ganglionic transmission in the cat. J Physiol (Lond) 220:297–314

de Groat WC, Saum WR (1976) Synaptic transmission in parasympathetic ganglia in the urinary bladder of the cat. J Physiol (Lond) 256:137–158

Delaere KPJ, Michiels HGE, Debruyne FMJ, Moonen WA (1977) Flavoxate hydrochloride in the treatment of detrusor instability. Urol Int 32:377–381

Delaere KPJ, Thomas CME, Moonen WA, Debruyne FMJ (1981) The value of intravesical prostaglandin E_2 and $F_{2\alpha}$ in women with abnormalities of bladder emptying. Br J Urol 53:306–309

Desmond AD, Bultitude MI, Hills NH, Shuttleworth KED (1980) Clinical experience with intravesical prostaglandin E_2. A prospective study of 36 patients. Br J Urol 52:357–366

Dhattiwala AS (1976) The effect of imipramine on isolated innervated guinea-pig and rat urinary bladder preparations. J Pharm Pharmacol 28:453–454

Diokno AC, Koppenhoefer R (1976) Bethanechol chloride in neurogenic bladder dysfunction. Urology 8:455–458

Diokno AC, Lapides J (1972) Oxybutynin: a new drug with analgesic and anticholinergic properties. J Urol 108:307–309

Diokno AC, Lapides J (1977) Action of oral and parenteral bethanechol on decompensated bladder. Urology 10:23–24

Diokno AC, Taub M (1975) Ephedrine in treatment of urinary incontinence. Urology 5:624–625

Diokno AC, Hyndman CW, Hardy DA, Lapides J (1972) Comparison of action of imipramine (Tofranil) and propantheline (Pro-Banthine) on detrusor contraction. J Urol 107:42–43

Donker PJ, Van der Sluis C (1976) Action of beta adrenergic blocking agents on the urethral pressure profile. Urol Int 31:6–12

Downie JW, Twiddy DAS, Awad SA (1977) Antimuscarinic and noncompetitive antagonist properties of dicyclomine hydrochloride in isolated human and rabbit bladder muscle. J Pharmacol Exp Ther 201:662–668

Duncan GW, Shahani BT, Young RR (1976) An evaluation of baclofen treatment for certain symptoms in patients with spinal cord lesions. Neurology 26:441–446

Ek A, Andersson K-E, Gullberg B, Ulmsten U (1978) The effects of long-term treatment with norephedrine on stress incontinence and urethral closure pressure profile. Scand J Urol Nephrol 12:105–110

Ekeland A, Sander S (1976) A urodynamic study of emepronium bromide in bladder dysfunction. Scand J Urol Nephrol 10:195–199

Ekman G, Andersson K-E, Rud T, Ulmsten U (1980) A double blind crossover study of the effects of terodiline in women with unstable bladder. Acta Pharmacol Toxicol 46 [Suppl] 1:39–43

Fingl E, Woodbury DM, (1975) General principles. In: Goodman L, Gilman A (eds) The pharmacological basis of therapeutics, 5th edn. Macmillan, New York, pp 1–46

Finkbeiner AE, Welch LT, Bissada NK (1978) Uropharmacology. IX. Direct acting smooth muscle stimulants and depressants. Urology 12:231–235

Fischer CP, Diokno A, Lapides J (1978) The anticholinergic effects of dicyclomine hydrochloride in uninhibited neurogenic bladder dysfunction. J Urol 120:328–329

Forman A, Andersson K-E, Henriksson L, Rud T, Ulmsten U (1978) Effects of nifedipine on the smooth muscle of the human urinary tract in-vitro and in-vivo. Acta Pharmacol Toxicol 43:111–118

Fossberg E, Beisland HO, Sander S (1981) Sensory urgency in females: treatment with phenylpropanolamine. Eur Urol 7:157–160

Fowler JE Jr (1981) Prospective study of intravesical dimethyl sulfoxide in the treatment of suspected early interstitial cystitis. Urology 18:21–26

Fox S, Krnjević K, Morris ME, Puil E, Werman R (1978) Action of baclofen on mammalian synaptic transmission. Neuroscience 3:495–515

Franz DN (1975) Drugs for Parkinson's disease: centrally acting muscle relaxants. In: Goodman
    LS, Gilman A (eds) The pharmacological basis of therapeutics, 5th edn. Macmillan, New York,
    pp 227–244
Fredericks CM, Green RL, Anderson GF (1978) Comparative in-vitro effects of imipramine,
    oxybutynin and flavoxate on rabbit detrusor. Urology 12:487–491
Gibaldi M, Grundhofer B (1975) Biopharmaceutic influences on the anticholinergic effects of
    propantheline. Clin Pharmacol Ther 18:457–461
Gibbon NOK (1965) Urinary incontinence in disorders of the nervous system. Br J Urol 37:624–632
Gleason DM, Reilly RJ, Bottaccini MR, Pierce MJ (1974) The urethral continence zone and its
    relation to stress incontinence. J Urol 112:81–88
Gosling JA, Dixon JS, Critchley HOD, Thompson S-A (1981) A comparative study of the human
    external sphincter and periurethral levator ani muscles. Br J Urol 53:35–41
Graham RM, Pettinger WA (1979) Prazosin. N Engl J Med 300:232–236
Hachen HJ, Krucker V (1977) Clinical and laboratory assessment of the efficacy of baclofen on
    urethral sphincter spasticity in patients with traumatic paraplegia. Eur Urol 3:237–240
Hackler RH, Broecker BH, Klein FA, Brady SM (1980) A clinical experience with dantrolene
    sodium for external urinary sphincter hypertonicity in spinal cord injured patients. J Urol
    124:78–81
Harris JD, Benson GS (1980) Effect of dantrolene sodium on canine bladder contractility. Urology
    16:229–231
Hartviksen K (1966) Discussion. Acta Neurol Scand 42 [Suppl] 20:180
Hebjørn S, Walter S (1978) Treatment of female incontinence with emepronium bromide. Urologia
    Int 33:120–129
Hebjørn S (1977) Treatment of detrusor hyperreflexia in multiple sclerosis. Urol Int 32:209–217
Hebjørn S, Andersen JT, Walter S, Dam AM (1976) Detrusor hyperreflexia. Scand J Urol Nephrol
    10:103–109
Hilton P, Stanton SL (1982) The use of desmopressin (DDAVP) in nocturnal urinary frequency in
    the female. Br J Urol 54:252–255
Hinman F (1974) Urinary tract damage in children who wet. Pediatrics 54:142–150
Hinman F Jn (1980) Syndromes of vesical incoordination. Urol Clin N Am 7:311–319
Hodgson BJ, Dumas S, Bolling DR, Heesch CM (1978) Effect of estrogen on sensitivity of rabbit
    bladder and urethra to phenylephrine. Invest Urol 16:67–69
Hollister LE (1978) Tricyclic antidepressants. N Engl J Med 299:1106–1109
Holmberg E, Waldeck B (1980) On the possible role of potassium ions in the action of terbutaline
    on skeletal muscle contractions. Acta Pharmacol Toxicol 46:141–149
Husted S, Andersson K-E, Sommer L, Østergaard JR (1980) Anticholinergic and calcium antagon-
    istic effects of terodiline in rabbit urinary bladder. Acta Pharmacol Toxicol 46 [Suppl] 1:20–30
Innes IR, Nickerson M (1975) Atropine, scopolamine, and related antimuscarinic drugs. In:
    Goodman L, Gilman A (eds) The pharmacological basis of therapeutics, 5th edn. Macmillan,
    New York, pp 514–532
Jensen D Jr (1981) Pharmacological studies of the uninhibited neurogenic bladder. Acta Neurol
    Scand 64:175–195
Johns A, Tasker JJ, Johnson CE, Theman MA, Paton DM (1976) The mechanism of action of
    dicyclomine hydrochloride on rabbit detrusor muscle and vas deferens. Arch Int Pharmacodyn
    224:109–113
Johnston JH, Farkas A (1975) Congenital neuropathic bladder: practicalities and possibilities of
    conservational management. Urology 5:719–727
Jonas D, Linzbach P, Weber W (1979a) The use of midodrin in the treatment of ejaculation
    disorders following retroperitoneal lymphadenectomy. Eur Urol 5:184–187
Jonas U, Petri E, Kissal J (1979b) The effect of flavoxate on hyperactive detrusor muscle. Eur
    Urol 5: 106–108
Jones RF, Burke D, Marosszeky JE, Gillies JD (1970) A new agent for the control of spasticity.
    J Neurol Neurosurg Psychiatry 33:464–468
Kaneko S, Minami K, Yachiku S, Kurita T (1980) Bladder neck dysfunction. The effect of the
    alpha adrenergic blocking agent phentolamine on bladder neck dysfunction and a fluorescent
    histochemical study of bladder neck smooth muscle. Invest Urol 18:212–218
Kedia KR, Persky L (1981) Effect of phenoxybenzamine (Dibenzyline) on sexual function in man.
    Urology 18:620–622
Khanna OP (1976) Disorders of micturition: neuropharmacologic basis and results of drug therapy.
    Urology 8:316–328

Khanna OP, DiGregorio GJ, Barbieri EJ, McMichael RF, Ruch E (1979) In-vitro study of antispasmodic effects of dicyclomine hydrochloride on vesicourethral smooth muscle of guinea pig and rabbit. Urology 13:457–462

Khanna OP, Barbieri EJ, McMichael RF (1981) The effects of adrenergic agonists and antagonists on vesicourethral smooth muscle of rabbit. J Pharmacol Exp Ther 216:95–100

Kiesswetter H, Hennrich F, Englisch M (1983) Clinical and urodynamic assessment of pharmacologic therapy of stress incontinence. Urol Int 38:58–63

Kilbinger H, Weihrauch TR (1982) Drugs increasing gastrointestinal motility. Pharmacology 25:61–72

Kleeman FJ (1970) The physiology of the internal urinary sphincter. J Urol 104: 549–554

Koelle GB (1975) Parasympathomimetic agents. In: Goodman LS, Gilman A (eds) The pharmacological basis of therapeutics, 5th edn. Macmillan, New York, pp 467–476

Kohler FP, Morales PA (1968) Cystometric evaluation of flavoxate hydrochloride in normal and neurogenic bladders. J Urol 100:729–730

Korczyn AD, Kish I (1979) The mechanism of imipramine in enuresis nocturna. Clin Exp Pharmacol Physiol 6:31–35

Kosman ME (1978) Evaluation of a new antidiuretic agent, desmopressin acetate (DDAVP). JAMA 240:1896–1897

Krane RJ, Olsson CA (1973a) Phenoxybenzamine in neurogenic bladder dysfunction. I. A theory of micturition. J Urol 110:650–652

Krane RJ, Olsson CA (1973b) Phenoxybenzamine in neurogenic bladder dysfunction. II. Clinical considerations. J Urol 110:653–656

Krier J, Thor KB, De Groat WC (1979) Effects of clonidine on the lumbar sympathetic pathways to the large intestine and urinary bladder of the cat. Eur J Pharmacol 59:47–53

Kunin SA, Limbert DJ, Platzker ACG, McGinley J (1970) The efficacy of imipramine in the management of enuresis. J Urol 104:612–615

Lapides J (1964) Urecholine regimen for rehabilitating the atonic bladder. J Urol 91:658–659

Lapides J (1974) Neurogenic bladder: principles of treatment. Urol Clin N Am 1:81–97

Lapides J, Dodson A Jr (1953) Observations on effect of methantheline bromide in urological disturbances. Arch Surg 66:1–9

Lapides J, Friend CR, Ajemian EP, Sonda LP (1963) Comparison of action of oral and parenteral bethanechol chloride upon the urinary bladder. Invest Urol 1:94–97

Larsen J-J, Mortensen S (1978) Effect of ritodrine on the bladder capacity in unanaesthetized pigs. Acta Pharmacol Toxicol 43:405–408

Lee LW (1949) The clinical use of urecholine in dysfunctions of the bladder. J Urol 62:300–307

Levin RM, Shofer FS, Wein AJ (1980) Cholinergic, adrenergic and purinergic response of sequential strips of rabbit urinary bladder. J Pharmacol Exp Ther 212:536–540

Levin RM, Jacobowitz D, Wein AJ (1981) Autonomic innervation of rabbit urinary bladder following estrogen administration. Urology 17:449–453

Levin RM, Staskin D, Wein AJ (1982) The muscarinic cholinergic binding kinetics of the human urinary bladder. Neurol Urodynamics 1:221–225

Leyson FJ, Martin BF, Sporer A (1980) Baclofen in the treatment of detrusor–sphincter dyssynergia in spinal cord injury patients. J Urol 124: 82–84

Lish PM, Labudde JA, Peters EL, Robbins SI (1965) Oxybutynin: a musculotropic antispasmodic drug with moderate anticholinergic action. Arch Int Pharmacodyn 156:467–488

MacGregor RJ, Diokno AC (1981) The alpha adrenergic blocking action of prazosin hydrochloride on the canine urethra. Invest Urol 18:426–429

McGuire E (1979) Urethral sphincter mechanisms. Urol Clin N Am 6:39–49

McGuire EJ, Lytton B, Pepe V, Kohorn EI (1976) Stress urinary incontinence. Obstet Gynecol 47:255–264

McNally C (1982) Smith-Kline Company. Personal communication (letter)

Mahony DT, Laferte RO, Mahoney JE (1973) Observations on sphincter augmenting effect of imipramine in children with urinary incontinence. Urology 1:317–323

Månsson W, Sundin T, Gullberg B (1980) Evaluation of a synthetic vasopressin analogue for treatment of nocturia in benign prostatic hypertrophy. Scand J Urol Nephrol 14:139–141

Medical Letter (1980) Dimethyl sulfoxide (DMSO). Med Lett 22:94–95

Merrill DC, Rotta J (1974) A clinical evaluation of detrusor denervation supersensitivity using air cystometry. J Urol 111:27–30

Meyhoff HH, Nordling J (1981) Different cystometric types of deficient micturition reflex control in female urinary incontinence with special reference to the effect of parasympatholytic treatment. Br J Urol 53:129–133

Milner G, Hills NF (1968) A double-blind assessment of antidepressants in the treatment of 212 enuretic patients. Med J Aust I: 943–947

Mirakhur R, Dundee J (1980) Comparison of the effects of atropine and glycopyrrolate on various end organs. J R Soc Med 73:727–730

Mirakhur RK, Dundee JW, Jones CJ (1978) Evaluation of the anticholinergic actions of glycopyrronium bromide. Br J Clin Pharmacol 5:77–81

Moisey CU, Stephenson TP, Brendler CB (1980) The urodynamic and subjective results of treatment of detrusor instability with oxybutynin chloride. Br J Urol 52:472–475

Moncada S, Flower R, Vane J (1980) Prostaglandins, prostacyclin, and thromboxane A₂. In: Gilman AG, Goodman LS, Gilman A (eds) The pharmacological basis of therapeutics. Macmillan, New York, pp 668–681

Montague DK, Stewart BH (1979) Urethral pressure profiles before and after Ornade administration in patients with stress urinary incontinence. J Urol 122:198–199

Muller J, Schulze S (1980) Imipramine cardiotoxicity: an electrocardiographic and hemodynamic study in rabbits. Acta Pharmacol Toxicol 46:191–199

Murdock MM, Sax D, Krane RJ (1976) Use of dantrolene sodium in external sphincter spasm. Urology 8:133–137

Nanninga JB, Kaplan P, Lal S (1977) Effect of phentolamine on perineal muscle EMG activity in paraplegia. Br J Urol 49:537–539

Noack CH (1964) Enuresis nocturna: a long-term study of 44 children treated with imipramine hydrochloride (Tofranil) and other drugs. Med J Aust I: 191–194

Nordling J, Meyhoff HH, Christensen NJ (1979) Effects of clonidine (Catapresan) on urethral pressure. Invest Urol 16:289–291

Norlén L, Sundin T, Waagstein F (1978) Beta-adrenoceptor stimulation of the human urinary bladder in-vivo. Acta Pharmacol Toxicol 43 [Suppl II]: 26–30

Öbrink A, Bunne G (1978) The effect of alpha adrenergic stimulation in stress incontinence. Scand J Urol Nephrol 12:205–208

Olsson CA, Siroky MB, Krane RJ (1977) The phentolamine test in neurogenic bladder dysfunction. J Urol 117:481–485

Olsson OAT, Swanberg E, Svedinger I, Waldeck B (1979) Effects of β-adrenoceptor agonists on airway smooth muscle and on slow-contracting skeletal muscle: in-vitro and in-vivo results compared. Acta Pharmacol Toxicol 44:272–276

Olubadewo JO (1980) The effect of imipramine on rat detrusor muscle contractility. Arch Int Pharmacodyn 245:84–94

Palmer JH, Worth PH, Exton-Smith AN (1981) Flunarizine: a once daily therapy for urinary incontinence. Lancet III: 279–281

Paulson DF (1978) Oxybutynin chloride in control of post-transurethral vesical pain and spasm. Urology 11:237–238

Pederson E, Grynderup V (1966) Clinical pharmacology of the neurogenic bladder. Acta Neurol Scand (Suppl) 42:111

Perera GLS, Ritch AES, Hall MRP (1982) The lack of effect of intramuscular emepronium bromide for urinary incontinence. Br J Urol 54:259–260

Perlberg S, Caine M (1982) Adrenergic response of bladder muscle in prostatic obstruction. Urology 20:524–527

Petersen KE, Andersen OO, Hansen T (1974) Mode of action and relative value of imipramine and similar drugs in the treatment of nocturnal enuresis. Eur J Clin Pharmacol 7:187–194

Petti TA, Law W (1981) Abrupt cessation of high dose imipramine therapy treatment in children. JAMA 246:768–769

Philp NH, Thomas DG (1980) The effect of distigmine bromide on voiding in male paraplegic patients with reflex micturition. Br J Urol 52:492–496

Philp NH, Thomas DG, Clarke SJ (1980) Drug effects on the voiding cystometrogram: a comparison of oral bethanechol and carbachol. Br J Urol 52:484–487

Raezer DM, Wein AJ, Jacobowitz D, Corriere JN Jr (1973) Autonomic innervation of canine urinary bladder: cholinergic and adrenergic contributions and interaction of sympathetic and parasympathetic nervous systems in bladder function. Urology 2:211–221

Raezer DM, Benson GS, Wein AJ, Duckett JW Jr (1977) The functional approach to the management of the pediatric neuropathic bladder. A clinical study. J Urol 117:649–654

Ramsden PD, Hindmarsh JR, Price DA, Yeates WK, Bowditch JDP (1982) DDAVP for adult enuresis – a preliminary report. Br J Urol 54:256–258

Rashbaum M, Mandelbaum CC (1948) Non-operative treatment of urinary incontinence in women. Am J Obstet Gynecol 56:777–780

Raz S, Caine M (1972) Adrenergic receptors in the female canine urethra. Invest Urol 9:319–323

Raz S, Smith RB (1976) External sphincter spasticity syndrome in female patients. J Urol 115:443–446

Raz S, Zeigler M, Caine (1973) The role of female hormones in stress incontinence. In: Proceedings of the 16th Congress of the Société International d'Urologie, Amsterdam, vol 2. Doin, Paris, pp 397–402

Raz S, Kaufman JJ, Ellison GW, Mayers LW (1977) Methyldopa in treatment of neurogenic bladder disorders. Urology 9:188–190

Rees DLP, Ransley PG (1980) Eskornade in the treatment of diurnal incontinence in children. Br J Urol 52:476–479

Rees DLP, Whitfield HN, Islam AKMS, Doyle PT, Mayo ME, Wickham JEA (1976) Urodynamic findings in adult females with frequency and dysuria. Br J Urol 47:853–860

Richelson E (1983) Antimuscarinic and other receptor blocking properties of antidepressants. Mayo Clin Proc 58:40–46

Richter JE, Castell DO (1982) Gastroesophageal reflux. Ann Int Med 97:93–103

Ritch AES, George CF, Castleden CM, Hall MRP (1977) A second look at emepronium bromide in urinary incontinence. Lancet I:504–506

Robinson AG (1976) DDAVP in the treatment of central diabetes insipidus. N Engl J Med 294:507–511

Rohner TJ, Hannigan JD, Sanford EJ (1978) Altered in-vitro adrenergic responses of dog detrusor muscle after chronic bladder outlet obstruction. Urology 11:357–361

Ron M, Shapiro A, Caine M (1980) The action of bromocriptine on human detrusor muscle. Urol Res 8:207–209

Rosenbaum AH, Maruta T, Richelson E (1979) Drugs that alter mood. Tricyclic agents and monoamine oxidase inhibitors. Mayo Clin Proc 54:335–344

Rossier AB, Fam BA, Lee IY, Sarkarati M, Evans DA (1982) Role of striated and smooth muscle components in the urethral pressure profile in traumatic neurogenic bladders: a neuropharmacological and urodynamic study. Preliminary report. J Urol 128:529–535

Roussan MS, Abramson AS, Levine SA, Feibel A (1975) Bladder training: its role in evaluating the effect of an antispasticity drug on voiding in patients with neurogenic bladder. Arch Phys Med Rehabil 56:463–468

Rud T (1980a) The effects of estrogens and gestagens on the urethral pressure profile in urinary continent and stress incontinent women. Acta Obstet Gynecol Scand 59:265–270

Rud T (1980b) Urethral pressure profile in continent women from childhood to old age. Acta Obstet Gynecol Scand 59:331–335

Rud T, Andersson K-E, Boye N, Ulmsten U (1980) Terodiline inhibition of human bladder contraction. Effects in vitro and in women with unstable bladder. Acta Pharmacol Toxicol 46 [Suppl] 1:31–38

Salmon UJ, Walter RI, Geist SH (1941) The use of estrogen in the treatment of dysuria and incontinence in post-menopausal women. Am J Obstet Gynecol 42:845–851

Schreiter F, Fuchs P, Stockamp K (1976) Estrogenic sensitivity of alpha receptors in the urethral musculature. Urol Int 31:13–19

Sjögren C, Andersson K-E (1979) Effects of cholinoceptor blocking drugs, adrenoceptor stimulants and calcium antagonists on the transmurally stimulated guinea pig urinary bladder in-vitro and in-vivo. Acta Pharmacol Toxicol 44:228–234

Smey P, King LR, Firlit CF (1980) Dysfunctional voiding in children secondary to internal sphincter dyssynergia: treatment with phenoxybenzamine. Urologic Clin N Am 7:337–347

Sonda LP, Gershon C, Diokno AC, Lapides J (1979) Further observations on the cystometric and uroflowmetric effects of bethanechol chloride on the human bladder. J Urol 122:775–777

Sporer A, Leyson JFJ, Martin BF (1978) Effects of bethanechol chloride on the external urethral sphincter in spinal cord injury patients. J Urol 120:62–66

Spyraki C, Fibiger HC (1980) Functional evidence for subsensitivity of noradrenergic α-2 receptors after chronic desipramine treatment. Life Sci 27:1863–1867

Stanton SL (1973) A comparison of emepronium bromide and flavoxate hydrochloride in the treatment of urinary incontinence. J Urol 110:529–532

Stanton SL (1978) Diseases of the urinary system. Drugs acting on the bladder and urethra. Br Med J I:1607–1608

Starr I, Ferguson LK (1940) Beta methylcholine urethane. Its action in various normal and abnormal conditions, especially postoperative urinary retention. Am J Med Sci 200:372–385

Stewart BH, Shirley SW (1976) Further experience with intravesical DMSO in the treatment of interstitial cystitis. J Urol 116:36–38

Stewart BH, Banowsky LHW, Montague DK (1976) Stress incontinence: conservative therapy with
   sympathomimetic drugs. J Urol 115:558–559
Stockamp K (1975) Treatment with phenoxybenzamine of upper urinary tract complications caused
   by intravesical obstruction. J Urol 113:128–131
Stockamp K, Schreiter F (1975) Alpha adrenolytic treatment of the congenital neuropathic bladder.
   Urol Int 30:33
Tulloch AGS, Creed KE (1979) A comparison between propantheline and imipramine on bladder
   and salivary gland function. Br J Urol 51:359–362
Turner-Warwick R (1979) A urodynamic review of bladder outlet obstruction in the male and its
   clinical implications. Urol Clin N Am 6:171–192
Turner-Warwick R, Whiteside CG, Worth PHL, Milroy EJG, Bates CP (1973) A urodynamic view
   of the clinical problems associated with bladder neck dysfunction and its treatment by endoscopic
   incision and transtrigonal posterior prostatectomy. Br J Urol 45:44–59
Ulmsten U, Andersson K-E, Persson CGA (1977) Diagnostic and therapeutic aspects of urge
   urinary incontinence in women. Urol Int 32:88–96
Ursillo RC (1967) Rationale for drug therapy in bladder dysfunction. In: Boyarsky S (ed) The
   neurogenic bladder. Williams & Wilkins, Baltimore, pp 187–190
Vaidyanathan S, Rao MS, Bapna BC, Chary KSN, Palaniswamy R (1980) Beta adrenergic activity
   in human proximal urethra: a study with terbutaline. J Urol 124:869–871
Veith RC, Raskind MA, Caldwell JH, Barnes RF, Gumbrecht G, Ritchie JL (1982) Cardiovascular
   effects of tricyclic antidepressants in depressed patients with chronic heart disease. N Engl J
   Med 306: 954–959
Walter S, Hansen J, Hansen L, Maegaard E, Meyhoff HH, Nordling J (1982) Urinary incontinence
   in old age. A controlled clinical trial of emepronium bromide. Br J Urol 54:249–251
Wein AJ (1979) Pharmacologic approaches to the management of neurogenic bladder dysfunction.
   Journal of Continuing Education in Urology 18(5):17–34
Wein AJ (1980) Pharmacology of the bladder and urethra. In: Stanton SL, Tanagho EA (eds)
   Surgery of female incontinence. Springer-Verlag, Berlin Heidelberg New York, pp 185–199
Wein AJ (1981) Classification of neurogenic voiding dysfunction. J Urol 125:605–609
Wein AJ, Raezer DM (1979) Physiology of micturition. In: Krane R, Siroky M (eds) Clinical
   neurology. Little, Brown & Co., Boston, pp 1–33
Wein AJ, Hanno PM, Dixon DO, Raezer DM, Benson GS (1978) The effect of oral bethanechol
   chloride on the cystometrogram of the normal adult male. J Urol 120:330–331
Wein AJ, Benson GS, Jacobowitz D (1979) Lack of evidence for adrenergic innervation of the
   external urethral sphincter. J Urol 121: 324–326
Wein AJ, Raezer DM, Malloy TR (1980a) Failure of the bethanechol supersensitivity test to predict
   improved voiding after subcutaneous bethanechol administration. J Urol 123:202–203
Wein AJ, Malloy TR, Shofer F, Raezer DM (1980b) The effects of bethanechol chloride on
   urodynamic parameters in normal women and in women with significant residual urine volumes.
   J Urol 124:397–399
Weiner N (1980a) Atropine, scopolamine and related antimuscarinic drugs. In: Gilman AG,
   Goodman LS, Gilman A (eds) The pharmacological basis of therapeutics. Macmillan, New
   York, pp 120–137
Weiner N (1980b) Norepinephrine, epinephrine and the sympathomimetic amines. In: Gilman AG,
   Goodman LS, Gilman A (eds) The pharmacological basis of therapeutics. Macmillan, New
   York, pp 138–175
Weiner N (1980c) Drugs that inhibit adrenergic nerves and block adrenergic receptors. In: Gilman
   AG, Goodman LS, Gilman A (eds) The pharmacological basis of therapeutics. Macmillan, New
   York, pp 176–210
Weinshilboum RM (1980) Antihypertensive drugs that alter adrenergic function. Mayo Clin Proc
   55:390–402
Whitfield HN, Doyle PT, Mayo ME, Poopalasingham N (1976) The effect of adrenergic blocking
   drugs on outflow resistance. Br J Urol 47:823–827
Woodhead DM, Hall TC, Snodgrass WT (1967) An effective control of benign enuresis. J Urol
   97:98–100
Yalla SV, Blunt KJ, Fam BA, Constantinople NL, Gittes RF (1977) Detrusor–urethral sphincter
   dyssynergia. J Urol 118:1026–1029
Ziegler MG, Lake CR, Williams AC, Teychenne PF, Shoulson I, Steinsland O (1979) Bromocriptine inhibits norepinephrine release. Clin Pharmacol Ther 25:137–142

Chapter 7

Pharmacological Treatment of Benign Prostatic Hypertrophy

Marco Caine

Introduction

In Chapter 1, when discussing the distribution of pharmacological receptors in the human urinary tract, it was pointed out that our studies on tissue removed during operations for benign enlargement of the prostate showed that there was a rich alpha-adrenergic receptor content in the enucleated hyperplastic tissue, and an even higher concentration of alpha-adrenergic receptors in the surgical capsule of the prostate. The beta-adrenergic receptor response in each of them was, for practical purposes, negligible (Caine et al. 1975). This academic finding ultimately led to the development of a pharmacological treatment for benign prostatic hypertrophy, which has gained increasing acceptance in recent years.

Rationale of Pharmacological Treatment

Structure of Prostate

It is worth stressing at the outset that, despite the fact that the prostate is usually thought of in terms of a glandular structure, it is in fact composed very largely of smooth muscle tissue. In recent years a number of stereometric analyses have been made of the various component tissues in the prostate, and Bartsch et al. (1979b), for instance, have shown that in the hyperplastic prostate the glandular epithelium constitutes only about 12% of the tissue, whereas the stromal tissue amounts to approximately 60%. Moreover, when the muscular tissue is compared with that of the normal gland, it is found not only to be hypertrophied (Fig. 7. 1), but on ultramicroscopic study there is evidence of

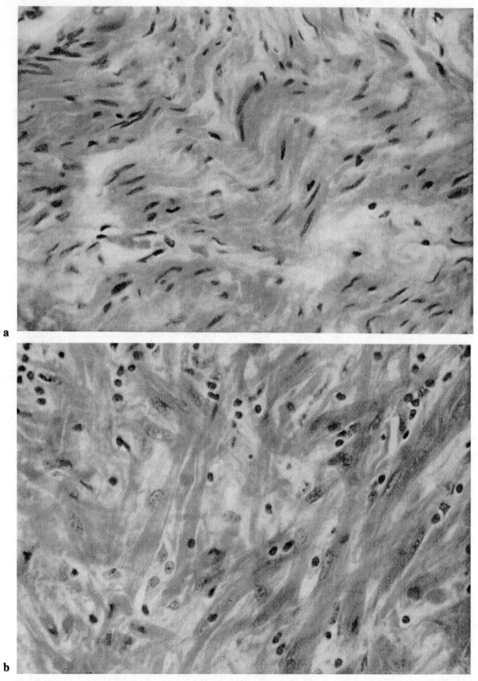

Fig. 7.1. Smooth muscle of prostate. **a** Normal prostate. **b** Benign hyperplasia, showing hyperplasia of the muscle fibres in the hyperplastic gland. ×40.

activation, with a three-fold increase in the organelles of the muscle cells (Bartsch et al. 1979a). In the surgical capsule of the prostate the glandular tissue is to a large extent atrophied by compression, and the relative proportion of muscular tissue is even greater. Since the urethra traverses the prostate a certain closure pressure is exerted on the walls of the prostatic urethra by the surrounding prostatic tissue, and it can be appreciated that variations in the tone of the smooth muscle in the prostate, both in the hyperplastic portion and in the capsule surrounding this, will produce variations in the closure pressure exerted on the prostatic urethra.

Effect of Sympathetic Stimulation on the Prostate

The primary effect of sympathetic stimulation on the normal prostate is to cause contraction of the intrinsic smooth muscle, via the alpha-adrenergic receptors that have been mentioned above. This will result in an emptying of the prostatic acini with expression of the prostatic secretion, as has been shown experimentally by Bruschini et al. (1978). More recently, Vaalasti et al. (1980) have shown in the rat that dilatation of prostatic glands occurs following peripheral sympathetic denervation with 6-hydroxydopamine, and they concluded that this dilatation was due to impairment of the normal emptying mechanism.

The above sympathetic effect relates essentially to acute activation of the sympathetic nervous supply to the prostate. However, less acute and more sustained variations in the degree of sympathetic stimulation will cause corresponding variations in the tone of the prostatic musculature. As explained below, these variations can be related to variations in the degree of obstruction and symptomatology in patients suffering from benign enlargement of the prostate.

Clinical Correlations

One of the typical characteristics of the symptomatology of benign prostatic obstruction is the fact that spontaneous variations can occur in the severity of the symptoms. It is well known to both patients and doctors that these can alter relatively rapidly, so that for example, at one period a patient may have very severe urgency and frequency of micturition, whereas a few days later this may become much less troublesome. Similarly, the force of the urinary stream and the degree of difficulty experienced in passing it can vary from time to time. Relatively little attention was paid to this phenomenon in the past, and no very satisfactory explanation for it was apparent. However, with the realisation that variations in sympathetic stimulation can result in variations in the degree of urethral obstruction produced, an explanation for the symptomatic variations becomes evident. This has given rise to the important concept that there exist two components in the urinary obstruction produced by benign enlargement of the prostate, which we have termed the mechanical component and the dynamic component.

Mechanical Component

The mechanical component consists of the basic underlying obstruction produced by the anatomical presence of the obstructing tissue, and as long as the amount and configuration of that tissue does not change, the degree of obstruction produced by it remains constant. In many cases, with the passage of time, this mechanical component will increase as the degree of prostatic enlargement increases, but this is normally a slow process measured in terms of months or years. On the other hand, spontaneous reduction in the prostatic size with diminution of the mechanical component of the obstruction does not occur.

Dynamic Component

In contrast to this, the dynamic component is related to the tone of the muscular tissue in both the hyperplastic prostate and the prostatic capsule, and will vary from time to time according to this tone, which in turn will vary according to the degree of sympathetic stimulation (Furuya et al. 1982). The obstructive effect of this component is additional to that produced by the mechanical component, and it can be understood that when the degree of sympathetic stimulation is at a minimum, the degree of obstruction will be that of the mechanical factor alone, whereas an increase in sympathetic stimulation and hence muscle tone will result in an additional degree of obstruction over and above that produced by the mechanical factor. Such variations in the level of sympathetic stimulation can occur spontaneously from day to day, and hence can explain the relatively rapid variations in the symptoms.

Blockade of the Dynamic Component

As a logical corollary of this concept, the idea emerged of abolishing or reducing to a minimum the dynamic component, by means of pharmacological blockade of the alpha-adrenergic receptors. It was anticipated that by so doing it might prove possible, in certain cases, to minimise the patient's symptoms. The degree to which the symptoms could be reduced would depend upon the underlying level of sympathetic stimulation, and hence the part played by the dynamic factor in the particular patient. Where this was basically high, or during a period of time in which it was increased, one could anticipate an appreciable improvement, whereas if the underlying sympathetic activity was already at a minimum, one could expect only a minimal improvement, or none at all.

Such pharmacological treatment by means of alpha-adrenergic blockers has now been in use for a number of years, and has proved to be effective and of considerable benefit in a large proportion of patients. The drug normally used for this purpose has been phenoxybenzamine (Dibenyline, Dibenzyline) which is effective orally, but on certain occasions where a particularly rapid effect is required phentolamine (Rogitine, Regitine) administered parenterally is an alternative possibility.

Actions of Alpha-Adrenergic Blockers in Benign Prostatic Hypertrophy

The action of phenoxybenzamine on the closure pressure of the prostatic urethra in the patient with benign prostatic obstruction has been investigated by a number of workers. Abrams et al. (1982a) performed urethral pressure profile recordings before and after administration of phenoxybenzamine, and showed a significant reduction in the height and area of the prostatic plateau following treatment. We have demonstrated the same effect on many occasions (Fig. 7.2). The diminution of the closure pressure in the prostatic urethra should logically result in an improvement in micturition, and the urinary flow rates were found to be significantly improved in a double-blind placebo-controlled series we investigated (Caine et al. 1978), as they were also in the series reported by Abrams et al. (1982a) and by Gerstenberg et al. (1980) (Fig. 7.3).

One of the interesting actions of phenoxybenzamine in these cases relates to the symptoms of frequency and urgency of micturition, and the often-associated detrusor instability. Whereas it was anticipated at the outset that alpha-adrenergic blockade would improve the obstructive urinary symptoms, the considerable improvement often encountered in the irritative symptoms was unexpected. Nonetheless, as detailed below, this is often an outstanding feature in the patient's improvement. The mechanism of this beneficial action is by no means

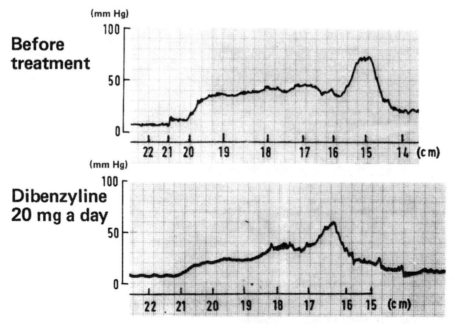

Fig. 7.2. Urethral pressure profile recording in a patient before and during treatment with phenoxybenzamine (Dibenzyline). Note reduction in height and area of prostatic plateau in latter.

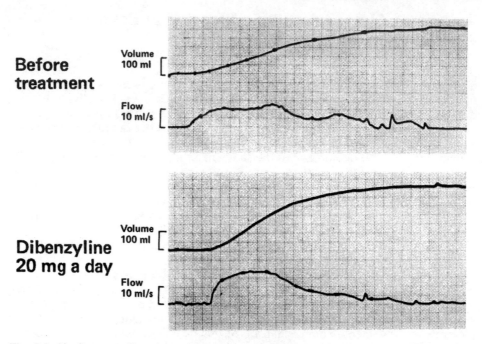

Fig. 7.3. Uroflow recordings in a patient before and during phenoxybenzamine (Dibenzyline) treatment. In the latter the maximal uroflow rate is almost doubled.

clear. It is difficult to relate it only to the diminution of the obstruction which originally produced these symptoms, for whereas the improvement following operative removal of the obstruction usually takes a few weeks, the improvement following phenoxybenzamine treatment may occur within a very few days.

One of the problems in understanding the effect of alpha blockers on the unstable detrusor is that the pathophysiological mechanism of this condition itself is not at all clear. It is possible that some light has been thrown on this problem by the experimental work of Rohner et al. (1978), and by our subsequent investigations (Perlberg and Caine 1982). Rohner showed that in the experimental animal, chronic obstruction of the bladder outflow can result in a change in the preponderant type of adrenergic response of the fundus of the bladder from beta to alpha, i.e. from relaxation to contraction. Our examinations of bladder fundus muscle removed at operation from patients suffering from prostatic obstruction showed a similar finding, and indicated a direct relationship between the presence of an unstable detrusor, irritative micturition symptoms, and an alpha-adrenergic response of the bladder dome in these patients. It is widely accepted that during the storage phase of the micturition cycle, whilst the bladder is filling, detrusor relaxation in the body of the bladder is mediated by inhibition of the parasympathetic activity together with a reciprocal sympathetic activity, the latter acting on the predominant beta-receptors in the bladder dome and enhancing relaxation. It can be appreciated that if the response of the detrusor alters from beta to alpha in its nature, instead of a relaxation of the detrusor during this phase an increase in tone could result,

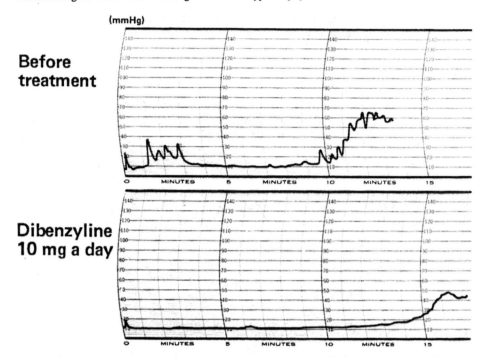

Fig. 7.4. Cystometrogram of a patient with prostatic obstruction and unstable detrusor. Filling with water at 25 ml/minute. The instability is abolished and the capacity increased when receiving phenoxybenzamine (Dibenzyline).

and it is possible that this could be associated with the phenomenon of detrusor instability and irritative micturition symptoms. In such a case, it would be understandable that blockade of these alpha receptors could counteract this instability and hence explain the beneficial effect of alpha-adrenergic blockers on the irritative symptoms.

We have found objective evidence of a reduction of unstable detrusor contractions on cystometrogram studies following administration of phenoxybenzamine (Fig. 7.4), and Gerstenberg et al. (1980) in a urodynamic investigation of 9 patients, reported a significant increase in bladder capacity and an improvement or abolition of bladder hyperreflexia in the 3 patients in whom it was present. Abrams et al. (1982a), on the other hand, were unable to confirm a significant effect on bladder instability in their cystometrographic studies.

Clinical Results

The pharmacological treatment of benign prostatic hyperplasia has now been in use for several years, and a number of publications relating to its clinical value have appeared. It must be remembered that, owing to the spontaneous variations that occur in the symptoms and the placebo effect produced by many medications, it is essential that properly controlled series be studied before it can be concluded that beneficial effects are indeed due to the drug under investigation.

In our double-blind placebo-controlled series referred to above, in addition to the significant improvement in flow rates, we found a statistically significant reduction in both diurnal and nocturnal frequency of micturition. We also found an improvement in obstructive symptoms experienced by patients, although this could not be quantitated satisfactorily. Despite the fact that clinically we had frequently observed an impressive reduction in residual urine following this treatment (Fig. 7.5), we were not able to show a statistically significant improvement in this respect, and concluded that this may have been due to the short period of observation used in this particular series, which did not allow sufficient time for the bladder to improve its emptying capability. In their controlled series, Abrams et al. (1982a) did find a reduction in residual urine, as well as an improvement in the obstructive symptoms of hesitancy and slow stream, although they were not able to confirm a significant improvement in frequency of micturition.

In addition to these controlled series, a number of other reports on the clinical results obtained with phenoxybenzamine have appeared in the literature. Kondo et al. (1978) reported an overall symptomatic improvement, including decreased frequency and easier voiding, in 42 out of their 46 cases (91%) who received the drug for periods of from 2 to 69 weeks. Waterfall and Williams (1980) investigated 20 patients, and found improvement in diurnal and nocturnal frequency, in the stream, and in the feeling of poor emptying, in from 76% to 85% of the patients. However, their series consisted of patients showing only 'minimal' prostatic enlargement, and the investigation was concerned more specifically with the improvement in opening of the bladder neck itself. Boreham et al. (1977) found an overall improvement in 18 of 27 patients (67%) completing a 7-day trial.

One of the largest series published to date appears to be ours, in which a review was made of 200 consecutive outpatients who received this treatment (Caine et al. 1981). This revealed an overall symptomatic improvement in 80% of the patients. Sixty-seven per cent of those suffering from diurnal frequency, 76% of those suffering from nocturnal frequency, and 79% of those with obstructive symptoms reported significant relief of their symptoms. Uroflowmetry was performed both before and after treatment in 102 patients in this series, and this showed an increase in the maximal uroflow of more than 50% in 72% of the cases, and of more than 100% in 46% of them. Although this particular series was not placebo-controlled, it should be noted that in our previous placebo-controlled series there were only 12% of those receiving the placebo in whom the maximal urinary flow rate was improved by more than 50%, and none at all in whom 100% improvement or more was obtained. The objective uroflow results in this series may therefore be regarded as highly significant.

From all the above reports, therefore, there seems to be no doubt that the use of phenoxybenzamine in patients with benign prostatic obstruction can afford both subjective and objective improvement in a large percentage of cases.

19.3.1973

1.4.1975

8.10.1975

Receiving
dibenzyline
10 mg a day

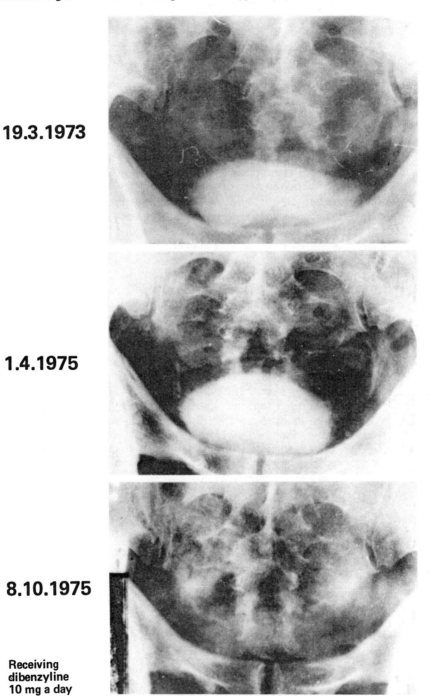

Fig. 7.5. Post-voiding bladder films in a prostatic patient show persistent residual urine over a 2-year period, abolished by administration of phenoxybenzamine (Dibenzyline). (Reproduced from *Eur Urol* (1977) vol 3, pp 1–6, by permission of S. Karger AG, Basle.)

Acute Retention

Causes of Acute Retention in Prostatic Patients

Acute retention in the prostatic patient is a subject of considerable interest. Although a certain number of these cases can be explained by progressive enlargement of the prostate which finally reaches the stage of complete obstruction, and others by the supervention of such complications as acute prostatitis or prostatic infarction, there remain a not-inconsiderable number of prostatic patients in whom there is no evidence of such complications and yet who develop a sudden acute retention, with very little warning or none at all. Moreover, in many of these cases the acute retention proves to be transient, and after decompression of the bladder the patient is once again able to pass urine as previously.

It is clear that such cases cannot readily be explained by changes in the mechanical component of the obstruction, but they are much more easily understandable in terms of a sudden variation in its dynamic component. More specifically, the occurrence of the retention could be explained by a sudden excessive increase in the tone of the prostatic muscle as the result of extreme sympathetic stimulation. This hypothesis fits well with the clinical observation that the administration of sympathetic agonists may result in acute retention in the prostatic patient. This is perhaps best known in the case of ephedrine, which is often incorporated in cough remedies in order to produce bronchial relaxation, and this effect was described as long ago as 1928 by Boston. Other adrenergic agonists such as phenylephrine, used in nasal drops, and phenylpropanolamine, used in cough medicines, have also been known to produce acute retention in the prostatic patient. Conditions which are known clinically to be liable to produce this effect, such as chilling of the body or overdistension of the bladder, are also associated with increased sympathetic activity in the body.

Urodynamic Findings in Acute Retention

Our studies of the urodynamic changes in patients during acute retention (Caine and Perlberg 1977) have shown that the maximal urethral closure pressure, and hence the site of maximal obstruction during such retention, is indeed in the prostatic portion of the urethra itself, and not at either the bladder neck or the pelvic floor. Both emptying the bladder and the administration of alpha-adrenergic blockers produce a reduction in the closure pressure in this region. We concluded from our studies that in certain of these cases, particularly those in which the retention proves to be transient, the initial stimulus causing the retention is sympathetic overactivity, and in the established condition this can be reinforced and the retention perpetuated by additional sympathetic stimulation together with a diminution in the contractile power of the bladder, both of these being due to the bladder overdistension.

The Place of Alpha Blockade in Acute Retention

According to this theory, it should be possible to influence certain cases of acute retention by the use of alpha-adrenergic blocking agents. These would be most likely to be effective when given in the initial stages of the development of retention, or if used prophylactically when acute retention is anticipated, but would be less likely to be effective once the retention is established and the secondary factors come into play. When wishing to obtain a very rapid action in order to abort an incipient attack of acute retention, it will be necessary to use a rapidly acting alpha blocker, and in this case the drug of choice will be phentolamine given intravenously. This has been used successfully in a number of our patients, and has therefore been of the greatest academic interest in supporting the above theory as to the underlying cause of the acute retention in these cases. However, the place for the clinical use of such a treatment is strictly limited, as many of the patients who fall into this group are, by virtue of their age and general condition, unsuitable for the rapid intravenous administration of an alpha blocking agent.

The prophylactic use is, however, of much greater practical value, and there are two groups of patients in which it is indicated. One group consists of those prostatic patients who suffer from repeated attacks of acute retention but otherwise often have only moderate prostatic symptomatology. These patients typically revert to their normal micturition each time the bladder is emptied, and then continue passing urine as before until the next episode of acute retention. These cases would appear, *par excellence*, to fall into the group of retentions due to sympathetic overactivity, and it has been found possible to prevent these recurrent retentions by use of a maintenance dose of phenoxybenzamine. This may be continued indefinitely in those patients in whom operation is deemed unneccessary, or may be used pending prostatectomy where this is decided upon.

The other group are those prostatic patients who have to undergo an intercurrent unrelated operation, for example a herniorrhaphy. It is well known that such patients, who may have relatively little trouble from their prostates whilst they are up and around and in whom there is no indication for prostatectomy, are particularly liable to develop an attack of acute retention immediately after the operation. This usually settles down satisfactorily after a period of catheter drainage, but it is obviously desirable to prevent it happening if possible. It has been shown that the prophylactic administration of phenoxybenzamine in these cases can very significantly reduce the incidence of post-operative retention of urine (Leventhal and Pfau 1978).

Indications for Pharmacological Treatment

From what has been written above, and from the detailed findings published in the papers referred to, it is evident that alpha-adrenergic blocking agents are effective in giving symptomatic relief and enabling freer and more effective bladder emptying in a large percentage of prostatic patients, as well as being of value in certain problems relating to acute retention in these patients. At the same time, it is evident from the discussion as to the mode of action, that these pharmacological agents in no way act upon the underlying mechanical factor, do not reduce the size of the prostate, and logically will not prevent further increase in the size of the prostate if this is destined to occur. In other words, it is clear that this treatment in no sense cures the underlying condition. What then, if any, is the place for such a treatment?

The answer to this must, to some extent, depend upon the attitude of the urologist to these cases. There are undoubtedly many cases of prostatic enlargement where operation is clearly and unequivocally indicated, and in such cases there can be no question of the pharmacological treatment coming in place of the necessary surgical treatment. On the other hand, there are large numbers of men who suffer from prostatic symptoms of a lesser or greater degree but in whom objective indications for operation are not present. If all such cases were inevitably progressive, there would be little to be gained by temporising, and one could justifiably take the attitude that all such patients should be operated on before their condition worsens. However, experience has shown that whereas some of these cases are indeed progressive, others are not and remain in a static condition for an indefinite time. Indeed, it is often stated that only about one third of patients suffering from prostatic symptoms will ever need an operation. A recent paper by Ball et al. (1981) is of considerable interest in this respect. In a review 5 years after initial examination of 107 patients with symptoms of prostatic obstruction who were not operated upon, they found that only 10 had required surgery whereas 97 had remained untreated. Although the patients in this latter group do not need operation from the point of view of danger, they are nonetheless suffering, and require relief for their symptoms.

In the past there was virtually nothing really effective that could be done to help these patients other than an operation, and many of them were subjected to surgery in order to give symptomatic relief. Nowadays the pharmacological treatment outlined above has proved to be the answer for many of these patients, especially those who cannot or do not wish to undergo an operation if it is not essential. With these facts in mind, and having regard to our review of 200 patients who received this treatment, the present indications for pharmacological treatment appear to be as set out in Table 7.1

Table 7.1. Indications for pharmacological treatment of benign prostatic obstruction

A. Symptomatic relief
    1. Patients not requiring operation
    2. Patients requiring operation
       Operation postponed for:
       (a) Medical reasons
       (b) Personal reasons
B. Conditions related to acute retention
    1. Prophylaxis of recurrent acute retentions
    2. Prophylaxis of retention following incidental operation
    3. Abortion of incipient acute retention
    4. To enable removal of catheter inserted for acute retention

Symptomatic Relief

The relief of micturition symptoms is undoubtedly the most frequent indication for the use of alpha-adrenergic blockers in the prostatic patient. The patients can be divided into two groups, namely those not needing operation and those who do require operation.

Patients Not Needing Operation

Patients not needing operation comprise the larger group, and as already indicated one can expect alpha-adrenergic blockers to provide relief of symptoms in approximately 70%–75% of these patients. The degree to which the symptoms will respond depends upon the part played by the dynamic factor in the given patient, and will have to be assessed in relation to any side-effects the drug may produce (see below). Some patients will obtain minimal benefit, which does not merit continuation of the treatment. Others may obtain very substantial relief of their symptoms, whether irritative or obstructive, and derive great and continued benefit from the treatment. We now have many patients who have been receiving this treatment for a number of years, without any worsening of the underlying prostatic condition. However, it must be remembered that some patients do have progressive prostatic disease, and it is essential to keep all of these patients under regular follow-up supervision.

Patients Requiring Operation

There are many patients in whom prostatectomy is clearly indicated but is not urgent, and in whom it is decided to postpone the operation. This may be for a medical reason, for example following a myocardial infarction or some other severe intercurrent illness or operation, or it may be in accordance with the personal wishes of the patient, as for example to enable him to complete certain commitments or to reach retiring age. In many of these cases it may be desirable to alleviate the patient's symptoms during the waiting period until the operation, and the alpha-adrenergic blockers have frequently been found to be of considerable value for this purpose.

Relief or Prevention of Acute Retention

Reference has already been made to two of the uses of alpha blockers in this field, namely (1) the prevention of recurrent attacks of acute retention in the prostatic patient, and (2) the prevention of retention following incidental operations. They may also occasionally be of practical use in enabling one to abort an incipient acute retention if a rapidly acting blocker is used in the early stages, although as already explained this is probably more of academic interest than of practical value.

In addition to these, there is a further application that is related to acute retention, and which is of considerable practical importance. This concerns the removal of a catheter inserted because of acute retention. Although many patients will be able to start passing urine spontaneously after removal of a catheter introduced because of a sudden acute retention, there are others who will not. Where the retention has been due to an organic change in the mechanical factor, such as acute infection or prostatic infarction, it is unlikely that efforts to remove the catheter will be successful, but in those patients in whom the retention has been due to sympathetic overstimulation, and simple removal of the catheter alone has not succeeded, a certain percentage of success will be obtained by removal of the catheter after having previously commenced treatment with alpha blockers. In the series of 200 cases we reviewed, phenoxybenzamine had originally been used for this purpose in 42 cases, and in 36 of these (86%) it was possible to free the patient from his catheter. It is noteworthy that in 8 of these 36 successful patients, previous attempts to remove the catheter *without* the administration of phenoxybenzamine had been unsuccessful, thus indicating that in these patients at least, the phenoxybenzamine had been an effective treatment. It is the author's belief that such attempts to remove a catheter should not be employed if there is dilatation of the upper urinary tract or diminution of renal function, but in other cases successful removal of the catheter is highly desirable even if the patient requires prostatectomy, for this will enable the operation to be performed in a 'clean' field, without the increased risk of infection associated with the indwelling catheter. In addition, the patient himself will usually be more comfortable whilst awaiting operation if he does not need to have an indwelling catheter.

Dosage and Administration

The alpha-adrenergic blocker which has been in general use up to now is phenoxybenzamine. This is effective orally, and the usual dosage needed for the symptomatic treatment of the prostatic patient is 10–20 mg a day. The drug is administered by mouth, and is cumulative in the body over about a week. The dosage will need to be tailored to the individual patient according to his response on the one hand, and the development of any side-effects on the other. Some patients find satisfactory relief with as little as 5 mg a day, or 10 mg taken every second day, whereas others have taken as much as 30 and rarely even 40 mg a day with benefit and without side-effects. A recent short communication by Abrams et al. (1982b) showed that there was no significant difference in the improvements produced in a group of 34 patients by doses of 5 mg or 10 mg a day.

If side-effects are experienced, they often occur maximally a few hours after administration of the drugs when the level in the body reaches a peak, and in such cases it may help to restrict the dose to night-time. Otherwise, it is probably best divided into morning and evening doses. We now have many patients who have been receiving this therapy for a number of years, and it has been our custom to advise an intermittent rather than a non-stop treatment, in the belief that this may lessen any tendency there might be to develop tolerence or resistance to the drug. Accordingly, we advise the patient to take the drug for approximately 2 months at a time, followed by an interval before the next course for as long as the benefit obtained from the treatment persists. Because of the cumulative nature of the drug and its slow release from the receptors, this benefit often continues for 2 or even 3 weeks after stopping treatment, and only when the patient again feels a return or exacerbation of his symptoms is the treatment commenced again.

In those patients in whom the phenoxybenzamine is used to enable removal of an indwelling catheter, it is recommended to give 20 mg a day for a week before attempting the removal, in order to allow the drug to accumulate and reach its maximal effect. When used prophylactically to prevent post-operative retention in patients undergoing elective operations, it is probably advisable to commence administration a number of days before operation so as to reach a satisfactory level in the body, and then continue administration in the immediate post-operative period until the patient is judged to be out of danger from the point of view of retention.

Although phenoxybenzamine has been virtually the only alpha-adrenergic blocker used for oral therapy to date, it is quite possible that other drugs of the same class may come into use in the future, and may even be tailor-made for this purpose. There is experimental evidence that prazosin (Minipress) is an effective blocker of the alpha receptors in the canine urethra in vivo (MacGregor and Diokno 1981), and of the human prostate in vitro (Shapiro et al. 1981), and evidence of its clinical effectiveness in BPH (Hedlund et al. 1983). Insofar as it is a specific blocker of the postsynaptic receptors, there are theoretical advantages to its use as compared with phenoxybenzamine (see Chap. 1).

In the occasional patient in whom it is decided to attempt to abort the development of an acute retention in its early stages, the rapidly acting alpha blocker phentolamine will be the drug of choice. This will need to be given intravenously, should be well diluted, and administered slowly with the patient recumbent and with constant monitoring of the blood pressure and pulse rate. The amount given will depend upon the response of the patient, and in our experience has usually been found to be in the region of 10 mg. As already mentioned, the practical application of such treatment is very limited, but nonetheless it may occasionally be applicable, especially in the younger and fitter patient, and may prevent the necessity for insertion of a catheter.

Side-Effects and Dangers

As has already been intimated, side-effects due to administration of alpha-adrenergic blocking agents are not uncommon, and these consist of other manifestations of the same alpha-adrenergic blocking action elsewhere in the body. Most frequently there is a reduction in blood pressure, which may result in dizziness and tachycardia, especially if the patient suddenly rises from a recumbent position. A feeling of tiredness or weakness may be complained of, and sometimes there is stuffiness of the nose. Impaired ejaculation may be complained of by the younger patients, and this may be due either to retrograde ejaculation due to relaxation of the bladder neck, or to a true lack of ejaculation due to impairment of contraction of the musculature of the genital tract. Less commonly, other side-effects such as difficulty with visual accommodation, a feeling of nervousness or 'tension', or a dry mouth may be complained of. As all of these are other manifestations of the alpha-adrenergic blocking effect of

Table 7.2. Side-effects of phenoxybenzamine therapy

A. *Common*
   Dizziness
   Tachycardia
   Palpitations
   Tiredness
   Weakness
   Blocked nose
   Retrograde or absent ejaculation
B. *Uncommon*
   Fainting
   Visual accommodation difficulty
   'Nervousness', feeling of 'tension'
   Dry mouth
   Increased anginal pain

the drug on the body they are temporary, pass off once the treatment is stopped, and leave no permanent ill-effects (Table 7.2).

The frequency of side-effects reported in the various publications has been very similar, and in our series of 200 patients they occurred in 30%. It is important to note, however, that in two thirds of this 30% the side-effects were either so mild as not to interfere with the treatment, or could be reduced to tolerable levels by adjustment of the dose of the drug, and in only one third of them (i.e. 10% of the total) were they sufficiently troublesome to cause the patient to stop the treatment. As these side-effects are troublesome but not dangerous, the decision as to whether to continue treatment with or without modification of the dose, or to stop it, will depend in the individual case upon the amount of benefit experienced by the patient balanced against the amount of discomfort caused to him by the side-effects. In our experience many patients have elected to continue treatment despite the presence of side-effects, because of the relief afforded to their urinary symptoms.

It must be noted that, despite the fact that phenoxybenzamine has been in clinical use for about 30 years without any suggestion of long-term ill effects, questions have recently been raised about the possibility of its possessing a carcinogenic effect. Certain in vitro mutagenicity tests (the Ames test and the mouse-lymphoma assay) have given a positive result, whereas the in vivo micronucleus test was negative. No one is certain as to the clinical significance of these tests, and full formal carcinogenicity tests are now under way, but will take a considerable time to complete. At the time of writing, until the matter is cleared up, it would seem wise to avoid, wherever possible, prolonged use of phenoxybenzamine in young people or in pregnant women for such conditions as neuropathic dysfunction. On the other hand, it seems likely that the risk to a patient of prostatic age, if it exists at all, is probably negligible, and that it is justified to use it when the clinician judges that it is advisable for the patient.

Contraindications to Pharmacological Treatment

It has already been stressed that this type of treatment is not a substitute for operation where this is necessary. Although, as already indicated, it may be used temporarily in patients awaiting operation where the operation is not urgent, its use will clearly be contraindicated where urgent operation is required.

The presence of any suspicion of an impaired cerebral blood supply, as suggested by a previous cerebrovascular accident or by clinical evidence of cerebral or carotid arteriosclerosis, should be regarded as a contraindication to the use of this treatment. It is possible that in such a case a drop in blood pressure induced by the treatment might predispose to a cerebral thrombosis, and although no such case has been encountered it would seem wise to anticipate such a possibility, and avoid use of an alpha-adrenergic blocker in such cases.

Apart from this, there appears to be no true medical contraindication to the use of phenoxybenzamine. Although the contrary is sometimes stated, we have been advised by our cardiological colleagues that cardiovascular disease is not generally a contraindication to its use. On the contrary, we have frequently used it very early after an acute myocardial infarction in order to relieve the severe symptoms of a patient confined to bed, with considerable benefit to the patient and no ill-effects. We did encounter one patient in whom anginal pain appeared to be exacerbated by the treatment, and this condition may therefore constitute a relative contraindication in certain cases.

Perhaps the greatest danger of this treatment is the possibility of improper use, either in a patient needing operation or in a patient in whom a diagnosis of carcinoma of the prostate has been overlooked. This of course is not a criticism of the treatment, but underlines the necessity for proper examination and assessment of the patient before embarking upon therapy. It is important to warn the practitioner against automatic and indiscriminate use of this pharmacological therapy in patients complaining of prostatic symptoms, and to stress that it must be employed only after the patient has been referred to, and assessed by, a competent urologist.

References

Abrams PH, Shah PJR, Stone R, Choa RG (1982a) Bladder outflow obstruction treated with phenoxybenzamine. Br J Urol 54:527–530

Abrams PH, Hollister P, Lawrence J, Doyle PT, Sherwood T, Whitaker RH (1982b) Preliminary note. Br J Urol 54:530

Ball AJ, Feneley RCL, Abrams PH (1981) The natural history of untreated 'prostatism'. Br J Urol 53:613–616

Bartsch G, Frick J, Ruegg I, Bucher M, Holliger O, Oberholzer M, Rohr HP (1979a) Electron microscopic stereological analysis of the normal human prostate and of benign prostatic hyperplasia. J Urol 122:481–486

Bartsch G, Muller HR, Oberholzer M, Rohr HP (1979b) Light microscopic stereological analysis of the normal human prostate and of benign prostatic hyperplasia. J Urol 122:487–491

Boreham PF, Braithwaite P, Milewski P, Pearson H (1977) Alpha-adrenergic blockers in prostatism. Br J Surg 64:756–757

Boston LN (1928) Dysuria following ephedrine therapy. Med Rec 56:94–95

Bruschini H, Schmidt RA, Tanagho EA (1978) Neurological control of prostatic secretion in the dog. Invest Urol 15:288–290

Caine M, Perlberg S (1977) Dynamics of acute retention in prostatic patients and role of adrenergic receptors. Urology 9:399–403

Caine M, Raz S, Zeigler M (1975) Adrenergic and cholinergic receptors in the human prostate, prostatic capsule and bladder neck Br J Urol 47:193–202

Caine M, Perlberg S, Meretyk S (1978) A placebo-controlled double-blind study of the effect of phenoxybenzamine in benign prostatic obstruction. Br J Urol 50:551–554

Caine M, Perlberg S, Shapiro A (1981) Phenoxybenzamine for benign prostatic obstruction: review
    of 200 cases. Urology 17:542–546
Furuya S, Kumamoto Y, Yokoyama E, Tsukamoto T, Izumi T, Abiko Y (1982) Alpha-adrenergic
    activity and urethral pressure in prostatic zone in benign prostatic hypertrophy. J Urol
    128:836–839
Gerstenberg T, Blaabjerg J, Nielsen ML, Clausen S (1980) Phenoxybenzamine reduces bladder
    outlet obstruction in benign prostatic hyperplasia: a urodynamic investigation. Invest Urol
    18:29–31
Hedlund H, Andersson K-E, Ek A (1983) Effects of prazosin in patients with benign prostatic
    obstruction. J Urol 130:275–278
Kondo A, Narita H, Otani T, Kobayashi M, Takita T (1978) Urodynamic study of lower urinary
    tract. IV. Clinical application of alpha-adrenergic blocker for the treatment of benign prostatic
    hypertrophy and bladder neck contracture. Jap J Urol 69:1232–1240
Leventhal A, Pfau A (1978) Pharmacologic management of postoperative over-distension of the
    bladder. Surg Gynecol Obstet 146:347–348
MacGregor RJ, Diokno AC (1981) The alpha-adrenergic blocking action of prazosin hydrochloride
    on the canine urethra. Invest Urol 18:426–429
Perlberg S, Caine M (1982) Adrenergic response of bladder muscle in prostatic obstruction: its
    relation to detrusor instability. Urology 20:524–527
Rohner TJ, Hannigan JD, Sanford EJ (1978) Altered in-vitro adrenergic responses of dog detrusor
    muscle after chronic bladder outlet obstruction. Urology 11:357–361
Shapiro A, Mazouz B, Caine M (1981) The alpha-adrenergic blocking effect of prazosin on the
    human prostate. Urol Res 9:17–20
Vaalasti A, Alho A-M, Hervonen A (1980) Effect of sympathetic denervation with 6-hydroxydopa-
    mine on the ventral prostate of the rat. In: Autonomic innervation of the prostate, Acta
    Universitatis Temperensis Series A, vol 113, part V, pp 1–14
Waterfall NB, Williams G (1980) Effects of phenoxybenzamine on bladder neck opening. J R Soc
    Med 73:345–347

Chapter 8

The Use of Adrenocortical Steroids in Urology

Marco Caine

Introduction

The adrenocortical steroids are used for their anti-inflammatory effects in many clinical conditions, amongst which are included a number of urological diseases. The mechanism by which the glucocorticoids produce their effects on the inflammatory reaction is not clear. It has been suggested that they may stabilise the membrane of the lysosomes, thus decreasing the release of destructive enzymes and vasoactive kinins. This may inhibit the growth of new capillaries, and suppress the formation of fibroblasts. In addition to their anti-inflammatory effect, it has been suggested also that in some instances they may act by depressing an immune reaction, either by reducing the release of antigen or by interfering with the resultant immune response itself, and this explanation has been suggested for any beneficial effect observed in those urological conditions in which an auto-immune aetiology has been postulated, such as interstitial cystitis and Peyronie's disease. However, it must be confessed that the whole theoretical background to both the diseases and the therapy is at present extremely hypothetical.

In using the adrenocortical steroids, especially systemically and for any prolonged period, the possibility of side-effects and complications must always be borne in mind. These include in particular the activation or exacerbation of peptic ulcers or of infections, including tuberculosis; the development of osteoporosis; psychotic reactions; salt retention; hyperglycaemia; and the development of cushingoid changes. Such drawbacks and hazards have to be weighed carefully against the degree of suffering or danger associated with the disease being treated in each specific patient, particularly if prolonged treatment is contemplated.

There are, at present, a limited number of urological conditions for which treatment with the adrenocortical steroids is an accepted form of therapy, even if the efficacy of the treatment is questioned by some authorities. The use of these steroids in the treatment of each of these will be briefly reviewed in this chapter, without entering into any discussion as to the nature of the diseases themselves, and without dealing with any of the other treatments recommended for the conditions. As in the rest of this book, those diseases which fall within the province of the nephrologist and not the urologist, such as the parenchymatous kidney diseases, are excluded.

Disease Therapy

Idiopathic Retroperitoneal Fibrosis

A large proportion of the cases of idiopathic retroperitoneal fibrosis fall into the province of the urological surgeon because of the obstruction to the ureters that is produced. There seems to be little doubt that treatment of this condition with corticosteroids can be highly effective, and the present author has seen palpable masses, proved at operation and by histological examination to be due to this condition, disappear virtually completely with this therapy. Whether the action is anti-inflammatory or due to an effect on a postulated auto-immune mechanism, or perhaps both together, is not clear. It goes without saying that the diagnosis of true 'idiopathic' disease as opposed to secondary fibrosis due to other causes such as drugs, inflammatory lesions or malignancy must be firmly established before the treatment is instituted; this inevitably means that at least one ureter will have been explored and the fibrosis biopsied.

It has been suggested, and it would seem logical, that the treatment is most effective if given during the early stages of the disease when there are systemic signs of activity such as fever, a raised erythrocyte sedimentation rate, and weight loss, so that the dosage and duration of the therapy can to a large extent by guided by the response of these parameters to the treatment (Charlton 1968; Ross and Goldsmith 1971).

Sometimes it is possible to abort the developing ureteric obstruction and avoid operation altogether by prompt institution of treatment, and in other cases operation such as ureterolysis will still be necessary, and corticosteroids will be used as an adjuvant therapy. Wagenknecht and Hardy (1981), in reviewing a collected series of 185 primary idiopathic cases, found that corticosteroid therapy alone was of value in 93% of those cases presenting moderate upper tract dilatation. In the cases requiring operation, they concluded that long-term post-operative therapy reduced the incidence of recurrent ureteric obstruction five-fold (from 48% to 10%). Abercrombie and Vinnicombe (1980) found that steroids were effective in treating recurrent post-operative ureteric obstruction.

The drug is administered systemically, the choice usually being prednisolone, and the dosage is tailored to the individual patient. In most cases the starting dosage is from 20 to 40 mg a day, and this is subsequently reduced progressively over a period of weeks in accordance with the response obtained, as indicated by diminution of the systemic signs of activity and a reduction in the size of the local mass and in the degree of ureteric obstruction.

Interstitial Cystitis

In its classical form interstitial cystitis is associated with the so-called Hunner's ulcer, but it is now widely accepted that other forms exist without ulceration, though with histological evidence of chronic inflammatory changes in the bladder wall. Many types of treatment have been recommended for this troublesome condition, amongst which the corticosteroids have their supporters. Both local injections of steroids into the bladder wall and systemic treatment have been advocated. Oravisto et al. (1970) reported on their experience with local infiltration of the bladder wall with prednisolone, but their results were not very impressive. Guerrier et al. (1965) used prednisolone systemically in relatively high initial dosages of 20 mg three times a day by mouth, reducing gradually to a maintenance dosage of 5 mg twice a day. With this regime they found that 9 of 11 patients treated obtained complete relief of their pain, and all had some degree of improvement in their frequency of micturition. It sometimes took several months for objective cystoscopic improvement to occur, but this did so in 8 of their 11 patients, with complete healing of the bladder lesions in 5. Badenoch (1971) reviewed 56 personal cases, and was much impressed by the results obtained with the steroids. He used much smaller dosages, starting with 15 mg of oral prednisolone daily and rapidly reducing this over a period of 2 weeks to 5 mg a day, which he then continued indefinitely. He reported that 19 out of 25 patients had maintained relief with this regime. It must be noted, though, that others have been less impressed with the results.

It has been the present writer's experience that oral prednisolone has undoubtedly given at least some patients with histologically proven chronic interstitial cystitis, in whom all other generally accepted forms of treatment have failed to help, considerable relief of their pain and frequency, as well as objective improvement in bladder capacity and cystoscopic findings. We have generally started treatment with 30 mg a day, and started a gradual reduction of the dose only after some relief has been obtained. We have usually found that complete cessation of treatment results in recurrence or reactivation of the disease, and that it is necessary to continue indefinitely with a maintenance dosage of 5–10 mg a day.

Peyronie's Disease

Peyronie's disease is a particularly difficult condition for which to assess the results of any type of treatment, for there seems to be little doubt that spontaneous improvement or even complete recovery can occur. This fact was emphasised by Williams and Thomas (1968), who followed up for periods of up to 8 years, 12 patients who did not receive any treatment at all. They found that 9 of them improved, and 4 became completely cured with loss of pain, disappearance of the plaque, and re-straightening of the penis. This natural history of the disease must always be borne in mind when trying to assess the efficacy of any reputed treatment.

Most authors employing adrenocortical steroids have advocated their local injection into or around the plaques. It must be stressed that injection into the fibrous plaque itself is quite impracticable unless a powerful, metal syringe is used. It is usual to combine the injection with a local anaesthetic such as 1% procaine, and often with hyaluronidase in the hope of improving the local permeability of the tissues. Williams and Green (1980) used local injections of 2 mg triamcinolone hexacetonide for six injections at 6-weekly intervals, in a group of 42 patients in whom no spontaneous improvement had occurred in the year prior to treatment. Of this selected group they reported that 14 (33%) showed a complete recovery or 'marked improvement', and concluded that the young patient with the small plaque was the one most likely to obtain benefit. Chesney (1975), in reviewing a personal series of 250 patients, concluded that the immediate and late outcome of the disease was considerably improved by local injections of 1.5 ml Decadron (a buffered solution of dexamethasone sodium phosphate containing 4 mg/ml) together with 1 ml of 1% procaine, at 2-weekly intervals for a total of 12 injections. This form of treatment is certainly unpleasant for the patient, and despite reports such as the above our limited personal experience with the method has not convinced us that it is of any real benefit.

Urethral Strictures

Earlier attempts to influence urethral strictures by local endoscopic or percutaneous injections of steroids at the time of dilatations were not very impressive. More recently, with the renewed interest in transurethral urethrotomy performed under optical control, there appears to be some evidence that associated local steroid therapy can improve the results. Sachse (1978), who has done much to popularise the use of the visual urethrotome, uses local instillation of 5 ml Terracortril gel (containing oxytetracycline and hydrocortisone) following operation. Hradec et al. (1981) injected 1–2 ml of Kenalog (triamcinolone acetonide, 40 mg/ml) transurethrally into the region of the stricture either before or after cutting it, and reported that the incidence of recurrent stricture formation fell from 19.4% to 4.3%. Gaches et al. (1979) reported that local circumferential injections of 2–4 ml of 5 mg/ml triamcinolone acetonide into the strictured area prior to incision, benefited patients who had failed to respond to two previous urethrotomies. In view of the slow rate of development of some strictures it is probably early as yet to assess the true worth of this prophylactic use of the steroids.

Osteitis Pubis

Post-operative osteitis pubis is a self-limiting disease, but causes severe suffering to the patient during its active period, which typically lasts for several weeks. Although infected cases of osteomyelitis may occur, it is the non-infected osteitis pubis which is considered in the present context. The aetiology is still not clear, but it is most probably vascular in nature. There is good evidence that the corticosteroids can greatly relieve the patient's pain, sometimes within 2–3 days of commencing treatment. Local treatment by injection of 25–50 mg of hydrocortisone acetate into the region of the symphysis and the affected bone, repeated after a few days if necessary, has been recommended (Barzilay et al. 1957). It is suggested that this produces a more rapid response than does systemic treatment, as well as having the advantage of freedom from the generalised effects. However, systemic treatment is associated with much less discomfort for the patient than are local injections, and has also proved effective (Marshall et al. 1952; Thornley 1955).

Tuberculosis

The steroids are sometimes used as an adjunct to anti-tubercular chemotherapy, in an attempt to minimise the fibrosis which frequently occurs during the healing phase. This is of particular importance in the case of ureteric tuberculosis, where stricture formation and subsequent obstructive renal damage are not uncommon. It has been suggested that the streptomycin used in the chemotherapy may predispose to this fibrosis. However, the evidence for this is questionable, and it seems more likely that the increase in the number of cases seen with fibrosis requiring repair is merely an expression of the increase in the number of cases in whom healing of the tuberculous process is now attainable, thanks to modern chemotherapy.

A number of authors have reported apparent success with this treatment. Okoličány et al. (1963) recorded the disappearance of ureteric obstruction in 13 out of 14 patients treated with prednisolone for a period of 6 weeks at a commencing dosage of 40 mg daily. Horne and Tulloch (1975) obtained relief of ureteric obstruction in 21 of 29 patients (72%) treated with 20 mg prednisolone daily for a minimum of 10 weeks. On the other hand, other authors have not been so impressed with the results. Claridge (1970), who stated that the results may sometimes be exceptionally good provided that treatment is started early with initial dosages in the region of 20–30 mg prednisolone daily, nevertheless admits that more often the results are disappointing. Gow (1970) reported that he found no significant difference at all between two groups of patients, one of which had received corticosteroids while the other had not.

One of the difficulties in assessing the results is presumably due to the fact that ureteric obstruction which is seen before the commencement of, or in the early stages of, treatment may be due to oedema and inflammatory thickening only. This may resolve with the anti-tubercular treatment alone, and it is difficult if not impossible to differentiate this from the obstruction due to commencing fibrosis. It would seem extremely unlikely that the steroid therapy would have any beneficial effect on an established stricture. Such considerations make it difficult to assess the true value of the treatment, and its effectiveness remains a matter of opinion. In our personal experience we have certainly encountered cases where ureteric strictures have appeared or progressed despite prophylactic steroid therapy. Perhaps the correct approach at present is to use adjuvant corticosteroid therapy if any signs of ureteric obstruction are present or appear during chemotherapy, but to appreciate that this cannot be relied upon to be effective in all cases, and to maintain a careful follow-up on the degree of obstruction by means of repeated urograms or other appropriate examinations.

References

Abercombie GF, Vinnicombe J (1980) Retroperitoneal fibrosis: practical problems in management. Br J Urol 52:443–445

Badenoch AW (1971) Chronic interstitial cystitis. Br J Urol 43:718–721

Barzilay B, Katz J, Wiznitzer TL (1975) Osteitis pubis treated by local infiltration with hydrocortisone acetate. Urol Int 4:373–382

Charlton CAC (1968) The use of steroids in a form of retroperitoneal fibrosis. Proc R Soc Med 61:875–876
Chesney J (1975) Peyronie's disease. Br J Urol 47:209–218
Claridge M (1970) Ureteric obstruction in tuberculosis. Br J Urol 42:688–692
Gaches CGC, Ashken MH, Dunn M, Hammonds JC, Jenkins IL, Smith PJB (1979) The role of selective internal urethrotomy in the management of urethral stricture: a multi-centre evaluation. Br J Urol 51:579–583
Gow JG (1970) Discussion on urinary tract tuberculosis. Br J Urol 42:711
Guerrier HP, Roberts JBM, Slade N (1965) Anti-inflammatory agents in the management of interstitial cystitis. Br J Urol 37:88–92
Horne NW, Tulloch WS (1975) Conservative management of renal tuberculosis. Br J Urol 47:481–487
Hradec E, Jarolinn L, Petřik R (1981) Optical internal urethrotomy for strictures of the male urethra. Effect of local steroid injection. Eur Urol 7:165–168
Marshall VF, Whitmore WF Jr, Petro AT, Poppell JW, Grant RN, Rawson RW (1952) Osteitis pubis treated with adrenocorticotrophic hormone. J Urol 67:364–369
Oravisto KJ, Alfthan OS, Jokinen EJ (1970) Interstitial cystitis: clinical and immunological findings. Scand J Urol Nephrol 4:37–42
Okoličány O, Škutil V, Payer J (1963) Glukokortikoide in der Behandlung der Tuberkulose der Harnwege. Urol Int 16:158–170
Ross JC, Goldsmith HJ (1971) The combined surgical and medical treatment of retroperitoneal fibrosis. Br J Surg 58:422–427
Sachse H (1978) Die Sichturethrotomie mit scharfem Schnitt. Indikation, Technik, Ergebnisse. Urologe [A] 17:177–181
Thornley R (1955) Some uses of cortisone in urology, with special reference to osteitis pubis. Br J Urol 27:1–6
Wagenknecht LV, Hardy JC (1981) Value of various treatments for retroperitoneal fibrosis. Eur Urol 7:193–200
Williams G, Green NA (1980) The non-surgical treatment of Peyronie's disease. Br J Urol 52:392–395
Williams JL, Thomas GG (1968) The natural history of Peyronie's disease. Proc R Soc Med 61:876–877

Appendix. Common Proprietary Equivalents of Drugs Mentioned in the Text

In the majority of instances, the official names of drugs have been employed throughout the text. However, in practice the urologist will frequently come across drugs under their proprietary names, and their true nature may not be immediately apparent. In order to facilitate identification of the corresponding official names, the most commonly encountered proprietary names of the drugs mentioned in this book, together with their official equivalents, are listed.

Proprietary name	Official name
Adalat	Nifedipine
Aldomet	Methyldopa
Aldoril	Methyldopa
Allegron	Nortriptyline HCl
Allertab	Chlorpheniramine maleate
Anectine	Suxamethonium Cl, Succinylcholine Cl
Ansolysin	Pentolinium tartrate
Anthisan	Mepyramine maleate
Apodorm	Nitrazepam
Apresoline	Hydrallazine
Arfonad	Trimetaphan camsylate
Aventyl	Nortriptyline HCl
Banthine	Methantheline Br
Benadryl	Diphenhydramine HCl
Bentyl	Dicyclomine HCl
Bicor	Terodiline HCl
Bretylate	Bretylium tosylate
Brevital	Methohexitone
Bricanyl	Terbutaline sulphate
Brietal	Methohexitone
Brufen	Ibuprofen
Buscopan	Hyoscine butylbromide
Catapres	Clonidine HCl
Catapresan	Clonidine HCl
Cetiprin	Emepronium Br
Compazine	Prochlorperazine
Cordilox	Verapamil HCl
Cystospaz	Hyoscyamine

Proprietary name	*Official name*
Danatrol	Danazol
Danol	Danazol
Dantrium	Dantrolene Na
Darbid	Isopropamide iodide
Darenthin	Bretylium tosylate
DDAVP	Desmopressin
Decadron	Dexamethasone
Decicain	Amethocaine HCl
Deltacortril	Prednisolone
Demerol	Pethidine, meperidine
Deralin	Propranolol HCl
Dibenyline	Phenoxybenzamine HCl
Dibenzyline	Phenoxybenzamine HCl
Dilantin	Phenytoin Na, diphenylhydantoin Na
Disipal	Orphenadrine HCl
Ditropan	Oxybutynin HCl
Dixarit	Clonidine HCl
DMSO	Dimethyl sulphoxide
Dolantin	Pethidine, meperidine
Dolestin	Pethidine, meperidine
Doryl	Carbachol
Duvadilan	Isoxsuprine HCl
Dyspas	Dicyclomine HCl
Epanutin	Phenytoin Na, diphenylhydantoin Na
Eskornade	Contains: phenylpropanolamine HCl, isopropamide iodide and diphenylpyraline HCl
Esracaine	Lignocaine
Flaxedil	Gallamine triethiodide
Fluothane	Halothane
Froben	Flurbiprofen
Halodol	Haloperidol
Histadyl	Methapyrilene HCl
Hypovase	Prazosin HCl
Inderal	Propranolol HCl
Indocid	Indomethacin
Intraval Na	Thiopentone Na
Intropin	Dopamine HCl
Inversine	Mecamylamine HCl
Ismelin	Guanethidine monosulphate
Isophrin	Phenylephrine HCl
Isoptin	Verapamil
Isuprel	Isoprenaline HCl, isoproterenol HCl
Janimine	Imipramine HCl
Largactil	Chlorpromazine HCl
Ledercort	Triamcinolone
Librium	Chlordiazepoxide HCl
Lidocaine	Lignocaine

Proprietary name	*Official name*
Lioresal	Baclofen
Lopress	Hydrallazine
Marcain	Bupivacaine HCl
Mecholyl	Methacholine Cl
Mechothane	Bethanechol Cl
Mellaril, Melleril	Thioridazine HCl
Minipress	Prazosin HCl
Mistura C	Carbachol
Mistura D	Phenylephrine HCl
Mogadon	Nitrazepam
Myotonine Cl	Bethanechol Cl
Neophryn	Phenylephrine HCl
Neosynephrine	Phenylephrine HCl
Nipride	Sodium nitroprusside
Norisodrine	Isoprenaline HCl, isoproterenol HCl
Novalgin	Dipyrone
Omnopon	Papaveretum
Optalgin	Dipyrone
Ornade	Contains phenylpropanolamine, chlorpheniramine and isopropamide
Pamine	Methscopolamine Br, hyoscine methobromide
Pantocaine	Amethocaine HCl
Pantopon	Papaveretum
Paragone	Diethylaminoethyl benzilate methobromide
Parlodel	Bromocriptine mesylate
Pavulon	Pancuronium Br
Pentothal	Thiopentone Na
Pirtiton	Chlorpheniramine maleate
Pitocin	Oxytocin
Pontocaine	Amethocaine HCl
Pramine	Metoclopramide HCl
Premarin	Mixed conjugated oestrogens
Primperan	Metoclopramide HCl
Pro-Banthine	Propantheline Br
Propadrine	Phenylpropanolamine HCl
Prostigmin	Neostigmine Br
Pyribenzamine	Tripelennamine citrate
Regitine	Phentolamine HCl
Robinul	Glycopyrrolate, glycopyrronium Br
Rogitine	Phentolamine HCl
Scoline	Suxamethonium Cl, succinylcholine Cl
Serax	Oxazepam
Serenace	Haloperidol
Serenid	Oxazepam
Sermion	Nicergoline
Serpasil	Reserpine

Proprietary name	*Official name*
SK-Pramine	Imipramine HCl
Stemetil	Prochlorperazine
Sudafed	Pseudoephedrine HCl
Tetracaine	Amethocaine HCl
Thorazine	Chlorpromazine HCl
Tofranil	Imipramine HCl
Triominic	Contains: phenylpropanolamine HCl, mepyramine maleate and pheniramine maleate
Tyrimide	Isopropamide iodide
Ubretid	Distigmine Br
Urecholine	Bethanechol Cl
Urispas	Flavoxate HCl
Valium	Diazepam
Valpin	Anisotropine methylbromide, octatropine methylbromide
Vasoxine	Methoxamine HCl
Vasoxyl	Methoxamine HCl
Vegolysin	Hexamethonium
Ventolin	Salbutamol sulphate
Voltaren	Diclofenac Na
Xylocaine	Lignocaine
Xylotox	Lignocaine

Subject Index

of further interest

The Ureter

Edited by **H. Bergman,** Miami
2nd edition. 1981. 760 figures. XVIII, 780 pages.
ISBN 3-540-90561-8

"It has been 14 years since Dr. Bergman brought out his first edition
of **The Ureter.** In reading the second edition, it is obvious that
Bergman and his excellent selection of authors have detailed the
anatomy, physiology, and pathology sufficiently to merit calling the
ureter a specific, anatomic organ rather than a simple conduit
carrying urine from the kidney to the bladder ... this is an excellent
reference for the academic and practicing urologist, adequately
pointing out the immense amount of new information recently
acquired concerning these two 'simple' muscular tubes."

A.J.Thomas
JAMA

Male Reproductive Function and Semen

**Themes and Trends in Physiology, Biochemistry, and Investigative
Andrology**

By **T. Mann, C. Lutwak-Mann,** Cambridge

1981. 46 figures. XIV, 495 pages. ISBN 3-540-10383-X

"For many years the standard text on the biochemistry of semen
and the male reproductive tract has been that published by
Thaddeus Mann in 1964. The present book replaces it as the authoritative source of knowledge on these matters ... an essential
reference book for clinical, laboratory, and research workers
concerned with function and dysfunction of the male reproductive
system."

W. F. Hendry
British Journal of Hospital Medicine

Idiopathic Hydronephrosis

Edited by **P. H. O'Reilly,** Stockport, and **J. A. Gosling,** Manchester
Foreword by E. C. Edwards

1982. 87 figures. XII, 132 pages. ISBN 3-540-10937-4

"This small book is described in the Preface as growing out of and
representing an extension of a symposium held in September 1980.
It is clearly not a straight-forward conference proceedings and
thereby avoids some of the more serious drawbacks usually associated with such volumes ... a useful update for anyone working in
this field who was unfortunate enough to have missed the original
conference."

British Journal of Urology

Nephrology Forum

Edited by **J. J. Cohen,** Chicago, **J. T. Harrington,** Boston, and
J. P. Kassirer, Boston

1983. 53 figures. XI, 383 pages. ISBN 3-540-90764-5

"This book contains 16 selected installments from the monthly
'Nephrology Forum' in the authoritative journal **Kidney International.** Each 'forum' consists of a summary of an actual patient's
history followed by a review of clinicopathological correlations,
diagnostic features and therapeutic option ... contains a wealth of
useful information and is highly recommended for all doctors inter-
ested in renal disease."

R. van Zyl-Smit
South African Medical Journal

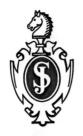

Springer-Verlag
Berlin
Heidelberg
New York
Tokyo

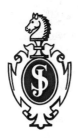